# Andrology Insights - Understanding Male Reproductive Health and Diseases

*Edited by Wei Wu*

Published in London, United Kingdom

Andrology Insights - Understanding Male Reproductive Health and Diseases
http://dx.doi.org/10.5772/intechopen.1004970
Edited by Wei Wu

Contributors
Abdoulie Dukureh, Balansama Marah, Behrouz Aflatoonian, Ekementeabasi Aniebo Umoh, Feng Pan, Feng Wu, Hale Bayram, Hongshan Ge, Jing Wei, Jinqi Ma, Jun Ye, Khawaja Raees Ahmad, Mahin Izadi, Marijan Kamilovski, Mohammad Ebrahim Rezvani, Peihao Wu, Qi Liu, Qiuqin Tang, Serajoddin Vahidi, Shaban Memeti, Sia Florence, Syeda Nadia Ahmad, Wei Wu, Xiaodong Liang, Yan Yuan, Yaprak Donmez Cakil, Ying Li, Yixuan Yan



First published in London, United Kingdom, 2025 by IntechOpen
IntechOpen is the global imprint of INTECHOPEN LIMITED, registered in England and Wales, registration number: 11086078, 167-169 Great Portland Street, London, W1W 5PF, United Kingdom

For EU product safety concerns: IN TECH d.o.o., Prolaz Marije Krucifikse Kozulić 3, 51000 Rijeka, Croatia, info@intechopen.com or visit our website at intechopen.com.

British Library Cataloguing-in-Publication Data
A catalogue record for this book is available from the British Library

Andrology Insights - Understanding Male Reproductive Health and Diseases
Edited by Wei Wu
p. cm.
Print ISBN 978-0-85014-820-6
Online ISBN 978-0-85014-819-0
eBook (PDF) ISBN 978-0-85014-821-3

# Meet the editor

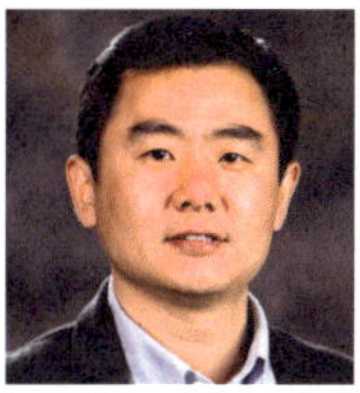

Dr. Wei Wu serves as Vice Dean of the School of International Education, Deputy Director of the Department of International Cooperation & Exchange, and Professor of the Department of Toxicology at Nanjing Medical University in China. He was a guest researcher at the National Institute of Environmental Health Sciences (NIEHS) between 2017 and 2018. He is the PI of the State Key Laboratory of Reproductive Medicine and Offspring Health, as well as the PI of the Key Laboratory of Modern Toxicology of the Ministry of Education. Dr. Wu is a member of several national and international societies focused on human reproduction and toxicology. He has also received multiple awards from many national societies for the originality and quality of his projects. Dr. Wu has authored 90 peer-reviewed papers in international journals. He has edited 8 books and collaborated on 10 books, 18 patents, and organized four international conferences. He is a reviewer for 110 international journals.

# Contents

# Preface

Infertility is a global health challenge affecting millions of couples worldwide, with male factors contributing to approximately 30% to 50% of these cases. This edited volume, *Andrology Insights – Understanding Male Reproductive Health and Diseases*, brings together a comprehensive collection of chapters that explore the multifaceted aspects of male reproductive health. This volume aims to provide researchers, clinicians, and students with an in-depth understanding of the biological mechanisms, diagnostic tools, and therapeutic strategies related to male infertility and reproductive disorders.

The volume begins with critically examining the impact of age on semen quality (Chapter 1), highlighting the physiological changes in male reproductive systems with advancing age and their implications for fertility. This chapter synthesizes evidence from human population studies, molecular research, and animal models to shed light on how paternal age influences sperm parameters such as concentration, motility, morphology, and DNA integrity.

Chapter 2, *Spermatogenesis*, delves into the intricate process of sperm production, detailing the stages of spermatocytogenesis, spermatogenesis, and spermiogenesis. The chapter explores the hormonal regulation, genetic factors, and external influences that alter spermatogenesis, providing insights into congenital disorders and idiopathic infertility.

The third chapter, *Natural Sperm Selection: Perspectives for More Successful Outcomes in ICSI*, shifts focus to assisted reproductive technologies (ART). It discusses the natural selection mechanisms that occur in the female reproductive tract and how biomimetic methods, such as microfluidic devices and chemotaxis-based techniques, can enhance sperm selection in ICSI procedures.

Chapter 4, *A Comparative Analysis of Gradient Centrifugation and Microfluidic Chips for Sperm Selection*, compares traditional density gradient centrifugation methods with emerging microfluidic technologies for sperm preparation. This chapter evaluates the advantages and limitations of each approach, emphasizing their clinical relevance in improving ART outcomes.

Chapter 5, *Detection and Clinical Application of Sperm DNA Fragmentation* addresses the growing importance of sperm DNA integrity in diagnosing male infertility. It reviews methods for assessing DNA fragmentation, such as the sperm chromatin structure assay (SCSA) and the comet assay, and discusses their clinical utility in predicting fertility outcomes and guiding therapeutic decisions.

Chapter 6, *Phytochemicals of Natural Fruit Extract Rehabilitate Male Reproductive Health*, explores the potential of medicinal fruit extracts to mitigate testicular damage caused by environmental toxins and insecticides. This chapter highlights the role of phytochemicals, such as antioxidants and phytosterols, in restoring sperm quality and testicular function.

The final chapter, *Cryptorchidism in Pediatrics and Adults*, examines the challenges posed by undescended testes across the lifespan. It discusses the embryological origins, clinical presentation, and management strategies for cryptorchidism, emphasizing the importance of early intervention to preserve fertility and reduce long-term risks such as testicular cancer and infertility.

This volume results from collaborative efforts by leading experts in the field of male reproductive health. I would like to express my sincere gratitude to all contributing authors for their dedication and insightful contributions. Special thanks are extended to the editorial team, whose meticulous work ensured the coherence and quality of this publication.

We hope this volume serves as a valuable resource for advancing knowledge and improving clinical practice in male reproductive medicine.

**Wei Wu**
School of Public Health,
Taizhou Clinical Medical College,
Nanjing Medical University,
Nanjing, China

Chapter 1

# Effect of Male Age on Semen Quality

*Abdoulie Dukureh, Sia Florence, Balansama Marah, Peihao Wu, Yan Yuan, Yixuan Yan, Feng Wu, Qi Liu, Ying Li, Jinqi Ma, Feng Pan, Jun Ye, Jing Wei, Hongshan Ge, Qiuqin Tang and Wei Wu*

## Abstract

Infertility is a global health problem that affects about 15% of couples of reproductive ages, and male factors contribute about 30–50% of these cases. Genetic and lifestyle factors were previously identified as causes of male infertility; however, idiopathic factors also account for about 30%. Interestingly, advanced paternal age has been identified as a factor responsible for poor sperm quality, which is also considered a factor responsible for male infertility. There are several changes in men's reproductive systems as they become older. Around 60, gonadotropin hormone levels rise, and testosterone levels fall, causing a decrease in testicular volume. This impacts Sertoli, Leydig, and germ cells. Aging also affects blood vessels, which may result in testicular fibrosis. Research indicates that males are more likely to develop benign prostatic hyperplasia, which can impair ejaculation and reduce semen volume. Many couples delay childbearing to their late 30s because of social and financial difficulties, especially in developed countries, which are considered until increased paternal age. The influence of advanced paternal age on sperm qualities is still debated. This review summarizes the evidence regarding the influence of age on semen quality parameters such as concentration, motility, morphology, DNA fragmentation, and total sperm count in human population, molecular, and animal studies. It will be helpful in the decision-making of the appropriate age of male childbearing.

**Keywords:** infertility, male, age, semen quality, reproduction

## 1. Introduction

Infertility is defined as a couple who cannot achieve a clinical pregnancy after 12 months of unprotected intercourse [1]. There is no data on the worldwide prevalence of infertility. Still, it is estimated that 15% of couples who are of reproductive age are affected by infertility, and male factors contribute 30–50% of these cases [2]. Infertility is a significant public health concern; approximately 15% of couples of reproductive age in the US use infertility services to achieve pregnancy [2]. In China, it has been approximated that the incidence of infertility reaches approximately

15–20% among women, accounting for an estimated 40–50 million individuals. At the same time, in men within the reproductive age bracket of 15–45 years, the prevalence stands at around 10–12%, encompassing approximately 45 million individuals [3].

Male infertility has a variety of etiological factors, ranging from genetic abnormalities and lifestyle choices to underlying medical disorders or drug use. Even though progress has been made in understanding the complexity of male infertility, idiopathic sperm abnormality has accounted for 30% [4]. While advanced maternal age has been found to affect pregnancy outcomes, such as spontaneous abortion, stillbirth, congenital abnormalities, and perinatal complications, some researchers have controversy on the effect of advanced paternal age on sperm quality [5]. Research shows that semen parameters are negatively affected by increased paternal age [6].

Aging is a physiological change that happens to our body naturally and is inevitable. Among the challenges that affect the male reproductive system during aging is a decrease in our reproductive capacity [7]. Recently, in many developed countries, men have postponed parenthood until their late thirties because of economic reasons, which raises a concern about advanced paternal age during the time of conception [8]. The percentage of men becoming fathers between the ages of 35 and 54 in the UK has surged by 15% compared to a decade ago [9]. Data from the United States reveals a substantive increase in the mean paternal age over the last 44 years (1972–2015), with an average increase of 3.5 years from 27.4 to 30.9 years of age [10]. In Denmark, the average age of fatherhood, which stood at 30.9 years in 1986, had increased to 33.4 years by 2016 [11]. Considering the fatherhood trend, researchers have brought attention to investigating the correlation between semen quality and age [12, 13]. There are different ways aging can affect men's reproductive organs. Testis volumes decrease at 60 years of age, testosterone decreases, and gonadotropin hormone levels increase with aging. It decreases Sertoli, Leydig, and germ cells. Aging affects blood vessels, which can lead to testicular fibrosis. Evidence shows that benign prostate hyperplasia incidents increase among aging men, which can have an effect on ejaculation and decrease semen volume [13, 14].

In addition to the typical factors contributing to male infertility, oxidative stress has emerged as a significant cause of age-related sperm dysfunction. As individuals age, the efficiency of mitochondrial function tends to decrease, leading to impaired electron transport chains and, subsequently, heightened electron leakage, resulting in oxidative stress.

Aging has been associated with increased oxidative stress levels, resulting in an elevated occurrence of lipid peroxidation and the generation of reactive oxygen species (ROS) within the mitochondria of sperm cells, which can alter sperm quality [7]. Therefore, male infertility has reached the young domain of men's health issues and imposed a tremendous public health concern as global sperm quality is dropping and the possibility that urologists and physicians will experience an increase in patients with problems with semen parameters [15]. Some authors suggested that sperm morphology is affected with increased age [16]. Aging has also been connected to decreases in daily sperm production, total sperm count, and sperm viability, as well as decreases in semen volume due to abnormal function of accessory glands [7].

This chapter aims to summarize the existing evidence regarding the influence of age on semen quality parameters, such as concentration, motility, morphology, DNA fragmentation, and total sperm count, in human population, molecular, and animal studies. By examining the available literature, this review will shed light on how age may impact various parameters of semen quality, including sperm count, motility, morphology, and DNA integrity.

## 2. Pathophysiology of age on semen quality

Given age-related changes in semen quality, two things need to be considered [2, 17]. First, cellular and physiological aging-related changes have been documented in various male reproductive organs, including the testicles, seminal vesicles, prostate, and epididymis. Autopsy studies on men who passed away from non-reproductive causes have revealed age-related phenomena such as the narrowing and sclerosis of the testicular tubular lumen, reduced spermatogenic activity, heightened degeneration of germ cells, and a decrease in the number and functionality of Leydig cells [18]. In the prostate, there is a reduction in smooth muscle mass and a decline in protein and water content. These changes may contribute to decreased semen volume and diminished sperm motility. Additionally, the epididymis, which is a hormonally sensitive tissue, can also undergo age-related alterations. This hormonal or epididymal senescence may lead to a decrease in sperm motility among older men. Second, as individuals age, they tend to experience more frequent exposure to external factors that can cause damage or result in diseases [2]. For instance, older men are more likely to have a more extended history of smoking compared to younger men. Additionally, they may have had previous episodes of urogenital infections or other health issues, further highlighting the cumulative effect of age-related exposures to potential risk factors.

## 3. Effects of advanced paternal age on semen composition and fertility

Semen is composed mainly of two elements: sperm and seminal fluids. Sperm originates from the seminiferous tubules in the testicles, while seminal fluids are produced in the accessory sex glands and excurrent ducts. Semen analysis evaluates these components, focusing on sperm count and semen volume [19].

Advanced paternal age (APA) demonstrates a notable decline in sperm parameters, such as semen volume, sperm count, motility, morphology, and viability. The direct link between male age and these variables remains unidentified, although numerous potential mechanisms known to be influenced by aging have been identified. These mechanisms include diminished functioning of reproductive accessory glands, cellular and physiological alterations characterized by reduced capacity to repair cellular and tissue damage, depletion of germ cells and androgen levels, and structural changes in the male reproductive anatomy, including narrowing of the seminiferous tubules, vascular insufficiency, and systemic diseases associated with the aging process [7, 20, 21]. Specifically, there is a decline in accessory gland secretions among elderly males, and there are distinguishable variations in both water and protein composition compared to their younger counterparts [2]. These are likely etiological cases, and the possible outcomes are discussed below.

### 3.1 Threshold of age

As previously mentioned, it has been reported that there is no alteration in sperm parameters until males reach the age of 34 years [2]. In a study conducted by Kidd et al., it was observed that the total sperm count was the initial parameter to be affected once an individual surpassed the threshold of 34 years. Subsequently, both sperm concentration and the percentage of sperm with normal morphology exhibited a decline at the age of 40 [2]. At the ages of 43 and 45, there were observed declines in sperm motility and semen ejaculate volume, respectively [22]. In a study conducted in China, the semen analysis of men aged 20–60 years was examined, revealing a negative correlation between age and progressive motility, vitality, and the percentage of normal sperm. Notably, the decline in rapid progressive motility and the rate of normal sperm morphology commenced gradually at 30, while progressive motility began to decrease at 40 [23]. The disparities in the findings among these studies may stem from variations in the study design, with differences in whether the studies were prospective or retrospective [24]. The discrepancies in findings across various studies may be attributed to differences in sexual abstinence time, study types (prospective or retrospective), distinct age groups, variations in sample sizes, diverse ethnicities, inherent biological variability, and the inherent limitation that semen parameters offer limited predictability of male fertility potential [25].

### 3.2 Semen analysis

Semen analysis holds a pivotal role within the spectrum of male fertility evaluation due to its capacity to comprehensively review testicular and epididymal functionality, nasal patency, and the performance of accessory sexual glands. Moreover, it plays a crucial role in evaluating sperm health to determine fertility potential [26] or in assessing the effectiveness of surgical interventions like vasectomy [27]. Semen analysis thoroughly examines various physical attributes of semen, such as color, odor, pH, viscosity, and liquefaction. It also assesses parameters like volume, concentration, morphology, sperm motility, and progression. These analyses are repeated at different intervals to ensure a comprehensive and accurate evaluation [28].

### 3.3 Kinematic movement of sperm

Computer-Assisted Sperm Analysis (CASA) enables the automated assessment of sperm motility, objectively evaluating diverse parameters that characterize specific kinematic aspects of sperm movement [29]. The CASA system differentiates and isolates each sperm in the microscope view, capturing a series of digital images illustrating the motion of sperm heads. This enables the reconstruction and monitoring of the unique paths taken by individual sperm [30]. Three sperm kinematic measurements (**Figure 1**), often used to characterize various aspects of sperm progressive motility, are the curvilinear velocity (VCL), straight-line velocity (VSL), and average-path velocity (VAP). VCL represents the time-average velocity (μm/s) of the sperm head's centroid along its curved path [31]. Veron et al. conducted a comprehensive cohort study involving a sample size of 5000 individuals. Their research examined the influence of age, clinical conditions, and lifestyle factors on routine semen parameters and sperm kinematics, specifically VSL, VCL, VAP, BCF, ALH, and MAD parameters. The findings of their study indicate a correlation between advancing age and decreased values in these parameters. These results suggest the presence of potential alterations in the molecular machinery responsible for sperm motility in individuals of higher age [11]. Similar findings were observed in a retrospective study involving 138 donors, where their sperm samples were analyzed using CASA. The study revealed that parameters such as ALH, VCL, LIN, and STR significantly decreased with age. However, no significant differences were observed among the groups regarding sperm concentration, proportion of motile sperm, and other kinetic parameters. These results further support the notion that age may impact specific sperm parameters related to motility [32]. A contradictory finding was discovered by Yanquan Li et al.,

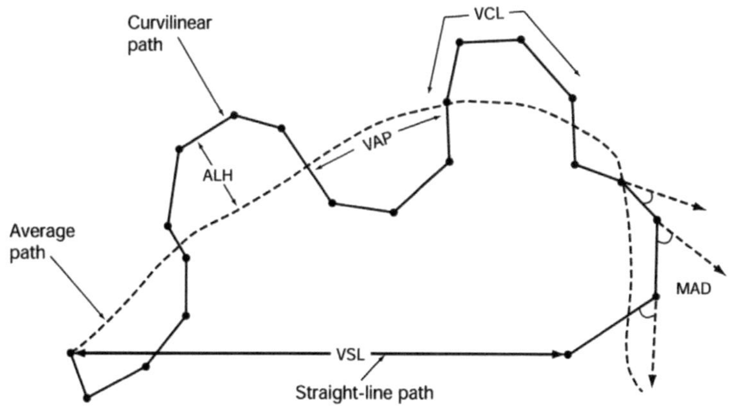


**Figure 1.**
*Computer-aided sperm analysis measures sperm kinematic parameters. VCL, curvilinear velocity; VSL, straight-line velocity; VAP, average path velocity; ALH, amplitude of lateral head displacement; and MAD, mean angular displacement. Adapted from the World Health Organization (2010).*

they found that VCL, VSL, and VAP are significantly increased over time. While VCL, VSL, and VAP significantly declined with age and abstinence time in a large cohort study of 49,819 using CASA [33]. This difference might be due to differences in the sample size and different lifestyle factors that are not controlled for, like healthy eating habits, smoking, and alcohol consumption. Still, all three of that research were done among healthy sperm donors, with the use of CASA and similar age groups from 18 years and above, which includes men in their 50s. Spermatozoa fertilization potential could be measured in ALH, VCL, and VSL [34]. However, tobacco use and heavy metals worsen VCL, STR, and ALH levels [26].

For many years, semen evaluation was considered the foremost laboratory test for male fertility [35]. Despite its critical role in male fertility assessment, standardizing semen evaluation remains challenging due to difficulties in maintaining sample quality and variability among laboratories. Consequently, establishing universally accepted protocols for semen analysis proves elusive in current research endeavors [36].

The World Health Organization (WHO) created the most often used reference values for human sperm and semen characteristics to assist in determining the reproductive status of men who are considering having children (usually a younger population) [37].

**Table 1** shows reference values for human semen according to the WHO editions (1999, 2010, and 2021). Observing the three other years in semen characteristics based on these standards, several trends and changes become apparent. There's a gradual decline in the recommended volume from ≥20 ml in 1999 to 1.4 ml in 2021, while sperm concentration in 1999 and 2010 had a threshold of ≥20 and 15 million sperm per milliliter, respectively; 2021 increased this to 16 million sperm per milliliter. A slight decrease in the recommended total motility percentage from ≥50% in 1999 to 42%, morphology remains consistent at 4% across all 3 years, and normozoospermic samples show a slight fluctuation, with 17.5% in 2010, dropping marginally to 16.0% in 2021. Overall, there's a noticeable shift in the criteria for normal semen parameters across the years, particularly concerning volume, sperm concentration, and total motility. Additionally, while some aspects show minor variations, others demonstrate more consistent standards over time.

| Semen characteristics | WHO 1999 | WHO 2010 | WHO 2021 |
|---|---|---|---|
| Volume (ml) | ≥2.0 | 1.5 | 1.4 |
| Sperm concentration ($10^6$/ml) | ≥20 | 15 | 16 |
| Total motility (%) | ≥50 | 40 | 42 |
| Normal morphology (%) | 14 | 4 | 4 |
| Normozoospermia | 31 (3.9%) | 138 (17.5%) | 126 (16.0%) |
| 1 semen abnormality | 217 (27.5%) | 269 (34.1%) | 257 (32.6%) |
| 2 semen abnormalities | 293 (37.2%) | 235 (29.8%) | 238 (30.2%) |
| 3 semen abnormalities | 247 (31.3%) | 146 (18.5%) | 167 (21.2%) |

**Table 1.**
*Evolution of semen characteristics: A comparative analysis across WHO guidelines (1999, 2010, 2021).*

This variance signals a concerning trend toward the global decline in sperm quality. According to the guidelines established by the WHO [38], a comprehensive assessment of sperm morphology should be conducted, encompassing a meticulous evaluation of various components, including the head, midpiece, and tail.

## 3.4 Semen quality

Semen quality plays a crucial role in male reproductive health and fertility. Recently, there has been an increasing focus on comprehending the diverse elements that affect semen quality. Of these elements, age has attracted noteworthy consideration owing to its possible impact on male reproductive health.

Semen quality is believed to provide information on male fecundity, defined as men's biological capacity for reproduction regardless of their wish for pregnancy intention [39]. It has been suggested that low semen quality may be a potential contributing factor in reducing fertility rates and increasing the number of children born after the use of assisted reproductive technology (ART) [40, 41]. There has been an ongoing debate about the decline of semen quality with age since 1982; many studies suggest a decrease in sperm quality in the general population, donors, or infertile men. Semen volume, the proportion of motile spermatozoa, and the proportion of normal morphology consistently declined with age among the basic semen parameters evaluated [42]. According to research, there are age ranges at which sperm quality starts to drop, with the earliest age range being 30–35 years old [22, 23].

The first step in the assessment of male infertility is a conventional semen analysis, which includes ejaculate volume, sperm concentration, motility, and morphology evaluated by the WHO accepted standards [2]. The decrement in comprehensive sperm quality attributed to advancing paternal age is intricately associated with alterations in testicular functionality, potential impairment resulting from urological disorders, and the influence of oxidative stress [43]. Common semen abnormalities encompass factors such as reduced semen volume (oligospermia, ≤1.5 ml), diminished sperm concentration (oligozoospermia, ≤15 million spermatozoa/ml), impaired sperm motility (asthenozoospermia, total motility ≤40% or < 32% progressive motile spermatozoa), and irregular sperm morphology (teratozoospermia, ≤4% standard forms). The severity of male infertility is typically categorized as severe when the sperm concentration is below 5 million per milliliter (severe oligozoospermia) or when sperm are absent in the ejaculate (azoospermia) [44].

## 4. Advanced paternal age (APA) consequences on fertility

Extensive empirical data underline the adverse effects associated with advanced maternal age, impacting both reproductive outcomes and fetal health [36]. A growing body of empirical evidence substantiates an age-dependent deterioration in sperm fitness. This observation assumes heightened importance given the escalating trend of delayed paternal age when initiating parenthood [16, 36, 45]. The exact mechanism responsible is not understood fully; literature suggests that APA could be accountable for having a negative effect on sperm quality [46].

According to Ford et al. [17], following adjustments for confounding variables, it becomes apparent that the probability of a fertile couple experiencing a time to conception exceeding 1 year significantly rises. Specifically, this probability increases from 8% when the male partner is below the age of 25 to 15% when he exceeds the age of 35. Consequently, it is imperative to recognize paternal age as an additional variable warranting consideration in the prognostic evaluation of infertile couples [17]. A similar study by Hassan and Killick stated that advanced male age is linked to a substantial decrease in fertility, with a significant increase in time to achieve paternity for men aged over 45 [47]. This effect remains independent of factors such as the woman's age, frequency of sexual intercourse, lifestyle, and other subfertility risk factors [47].

Increased sperm concentration and diploidy, as well as a decrease in semen volume and sperm vitality, are all linked to aging in infertile men. However, male age does not impact DNA fragmentation, shape, or motility [42]. Boitrelle et al. suggest that age-related changes in infertile men include an increase in sperm concentration and diploidy, as well as a decrease in semen volume and sperm vitality [4]. However, male age does not affect morphology, DNA fragmentation, or motility [42]. In a recent systematic review and meta-analysis, semen data from nearly 94,000 men across 90 studies were examined. The findings revealed a consistent age-related decrease in semen quality [16]. Age exhibited associations with slight to moderate declines in various semen parameters, including semen volume, total sperm count per ejaculate, percentage motility, progressive motility, and normal morphology.

Several researchers have identified an increase in paternal age correlates with spontaneous abortion [48]. The decline in semen quality is exacerbated by advancing age, academic achievement, and persistent tobacco use [49]. However, studies showed contradictory results. Sharma et al. stated in their studies that advanced paternal age is associated with increased DNA fragmentation in sperm, suggesting a potentially harmful effect on sperm quality [5]. Also, another study reported that advanced paternal age significantly correlates with decreased sperm motility, contradicting the claim that male age does not affect motility [6]. As couples delay childbearing, it is becoming essential to determine the association between paternal age, semen quality, and high risk of male infertility [50, 51]. The literature on the effect of paternal age on semen parameters is still controversial [52].

According to Wyrobek et al. [53], APA has been linked to conditions with intricate causes like schizophrenia, as well as to hereditary disorders that follow an autosomal dominant pattern, such as achondroplasia and Apert's syndrome. Their findings also suggest that as males progress through aging, their ability to achieve successful pregnancies declines, showing initial signs during their early reproductive years. Additionally, there is a heightened likelihood of them having children with achondroplasia mutations, as well as a variable risk of fathering offspring with Apert syndrome across different groups. However, there is no elevated chance of fathering offspring with aneuploid conditions like Down, Klinefelter, Turner, triple X, XYY syndromes, or triploid embryos [54]. It is consistently documented in the literature that advanced paternal age is consistently linked to an extended duration for achieving pregnancy and reduced probability of conception, persisting even after accounting for the age of the female partner through appropriate adjustments; notably, in couples receiving ART, a meta-analysis also suggested a deleterious effect of increasing male age on the outcome of ART, with clinical pregnancy rates and live birth rates found to be significantly decreased when male age was >40 years [53]. Elevated paternal age (45 years or above) is connected to an escalated likelihood of preterm birth, infants born with low birth weight, and infants exhibiting low Apgar scores [55]. It also likely amplifies potential maternal ramifications, including a heightened risk of pre-eclampsia and gestational diabetes [45].

## 5. Influence of age on sperm parameters

### 5.1 Effect of aging on sperm count

Sperm count or the number of sperm cells present in a given semen sample, is a crucial indicator of male fertility. Studies have sought to unravel the relationship between advancing age and sperm count, with compelling evidence indicating a gradual decline in sperm count as men grow older. Levitas et al. conducted an extensive study on men attending a fertility center and reported a significant inverse correlation between age and sperm concentration [56]. This finding was echoed in a comprehensive meta-analysis by Johnson et al., which synthesized data from various populations and confirmed a statistically significant decrease in sperm count with increasing age [16].

A comprehensive meta-analysis by Levine et al. encompassing data from over 42,000 men reported a consistent decline in sperm counts across different age groups. The study concluded that sperm counts have significantly decreased over the past few decades, with a 50–60% reduction in total sperm count among men in Western countries. This decline was more pronounced in older age groups [15].

The age-related decline in sperm count is intricately linked to hormonal and physiological changes in the male reproductive system over time. Cooper et al. elucidated that aging is associated with diminished levels of testosterone and an elevation in follicle-stimulating hormone (FSH), both of which are pivotal in regulating spermatogenesis [57]. This hormonal shift is postulated to contribute to reduced sperm production and lower sperm count.

Aging is also accompanied by heightened oxidative stress, a phenomenon implicated in the age-related decline of various physiological functions. Bui et al. [40] discussed how oxidative stress can result in DNA damage within sperm cells, leading to impaired sperm quality and potentially reduced sperm count. This oxidative stress-induced damage to sperm DNA can result in compromised sperm function and further exacerbate the age-associated decrease in sperm count.

### 5.2 Effect of aging on sperm motility

Sperm motility, the ability of sperm to move efficiently, is another essential factor affecting fertility. Research indicates a significant relationship between age and sperm motility. A study by Kidd et al. [2] observed that sperm motility decreases progressively with age, particularly after age 50. The decline in motility could be attributed to changes in the structure and function of the male reproductive system, including decreased testosterone levels and alterations in the epididymis, where sperm mature and gain their motility. Stone et al. [22] identified an age threshold of >45 years for sperm concentration and motility reduction. Another study done by Stone et al. [40] also found a similar age bracket in which sperm motility decreased after 43 years [58]. It was discovered that sperm motility appears to be the parameter most notably influenced by age, as individuals across all age groups demonstrated a significantly heightened susceptibility to experiencing atypical results compared to males aged 21–30 years. It is noteworthy that spermatozoa acquire their motility within the prostate and epididymis. Consequently, the observed decline in motility associated with aging can be attributed to the progressive deterioration in endocrine function that individuals undergo as they age.

### 5.3 Effect of aging on sperm morphology

Sperm morphology refers to the size and shape of sperm cells, and abnormal morphology can hinder fertilization; for the sperm cell to be considered morphologically normal, a spermatozoon must precisely conform to strict criteria regarding the size and shape of its entire structure, including the head, midpiece, and tail [59]. The characterization of morphologically normal sperm, capable of fertilization, was established by examining spermatozoa retrieved from the female genital tract, notably from post-coital endocervical mucus and the surface of the zona pellucida. Morphogenetic alterations in human spermatozoa occurring during spermatogenesis or epididymal maturation can lead to imperfections and anomalies, resulting in the generation of spermatozoa displaying diverse abnormal forms. These anomalies can be detected through routine semen analysis [60]. Hence, aging may directly impact testicular and epididymal function, potentially resulting in abnormal sperm morphology [7].

Several studies have investigated the connection between age and sperm morphology. Research indicates that there may be an annual decrease in the average sperm shape of 0.2–0.9%, which might lead to a fall in normal morphology of 4–18% over 20 years [7, 61]. Another study proposed that oxidative stress and cumulative DNA damage might contribute to these age-related changes in sperm morphology [62]. Due to differences in the morphology criteria used by different researchers, it is essential to acknowledge the limitations when comparing sperm morphology data across studies.

### 5.4 Effect of aging on sperm concentration

In the absence of confounding variables, male aging exhibited a statistically significant correlation with a decline in both sperm concentration and motility, alongside an observable elevation in the occurrence of sperm necrosis [63]. As the patient's age increased, there was a gradual reduction in sperm concentration ($P = 0.046$). Shindel et al. concluded in their research a discernible trend wherein the sperm concentration experiences a slight decline in tandem with the progression of patient age [34].

Research conducted by Smith et al. demonstrated a negative correlation between age and sperm concentration, revealing that older men tend to exhibit lower sperm concentrations compared to their younger counterparts [64]. This finding was consistent with a meta-analysis by Levista et al. in 2007, which synthesized data from various studies to confirm a statistically significant decline in sperm concentration with increasing age [57]. Aging influences testicular function and hormone levels, potentially contributing to the observed decrease in sperm concentration. The study by Cooper et al. highlighted that older men often experience reduced levels of testosterone and an increase in circulating follicle-stimulating hormone (FSH), which could play a role in diminishing sperm production [57].

Additionally, oxidative stress, exacerbated by aging, has been implicated as a potential mechanism underlying the decline in sperm concentration. As discussed by Agarwal et al., oxidative stress can contribute to DNA damage within sperm cells, resulting in decreased [65].

Moreover, lifestyle factors, such as smoking, alcohol consumption, and obesity, which often accumulate over time, can contribute to the deterioration of sperm concentration in older individuals [66]. These factors can negatively impact sperm production, motility, and morphology, compounding the age-related decline in sperm quality and concentration. Another study reported a decrease in sperm concentration by approximately 3.3% for each year of advancing age, resulting in a cumulative decrease of roughly 66% in concentration between the ages of 30 and 50 [60].

### 5.5 Effect of aging on sperm DNA integrity

Maintaining DNA integrity in sperm cells is vital to ensure healthy embryo development. Age-related factors such as increased DNA fragmentation have been associated with male aging, evidenced by previous studies that found a positive correlation between age and DNA fragmentation in sperm cells. The study postulated that accumulating oxidative stress and environmental exposures over time could contribute to DNA damage. This damage may lead to impaired fertility and an increased risk of miscarriages and congenital disabilities [67].

The impact of a man's age on the level of DNA damage in his sperm has notable implications for individuals seeking fertility treatment. However, there are worries regarding the potential transfer of this damaged DNA to the offspring, significantly when the extent of damage surpasses the oocyte's ability to repair it [68]. Plastira et al. reveal a correlation between advancing age and a diminishing trend in conventional semen parameters. Additionally, an escalation in human sperm DNA damage and compromised chromatin packaging are observed, particularly among patients diagnosed with oligo-astheno-terato-zoo-spermia who are above the age of 35 [69] in a comprehensive investigation encompassing both fertile and infertile male cohorts, Moskovtsev and colleagues documented a notable elevation in DNA fragmentation levels among individuals aged above 45 years. Specifically, the percentage index denoting DNA fragmentation exhibited a two-fold increase in men over 45 years in contrast to their counterparts below the age of 30 years [70]. Singh et al. observed a substantial rise in the proportion of sperm exhibiting extensive DNA damage among individuals aged 36–57 years compared to those within the 20–35-year age bracket. Additionally, their findings unveiled a gradual reduction in sperm apoptosis linked to advancing age. The researchers postulated that the escalated sperm DNA damage associated with increasing age might be attributed to a diminished efficacy of sperm selection processes occurring with aging [68]. Conversely, Nijs et al. and colleagues conducted an investigation involving couples undergoing in vitro fertilization (IVF) and concluded that there exists no significant correlation between advanced paternal age and sperm DNA damage [71].

A previous cohort study comprising 1974 normozoospermic men undergoing evaluation for infertility reported that 11% of these individuals exhibit notable levels of sperm DNA fragmentation [20]. Furthermore, their findings establish a correlation between the degree of DNA fragmentation, sperm motility, and the father's age. According to Colin et al., a discernible pattern emerged wherein higher levels of DNA fragmentation were evident in the elder cohorts. The age at which these findings became prominent was around 40 years. Progressive male aging demonstrated a favorable association with elevated levels of follicle-stimulating hormone (FSH) and sex hormone-binding globulin (SHBG) while exhibiting an adverse correlation with sperm concentration [72].

### 5.6 Effect of aging on semen volume

Semen volume has been suggested as an early indicator of poor semen quality, even preceding the identification of abnormalities in sperm concentration, motility, and morphology [73]. Additionally, it can determine the secretory functions of accessory glands, particularly the seminal vesicles [73].

Despite numerous studies indicating a negative relationship between age and semen volume, there remains a lack of agreement among researchers on this matter. In a comprehensive analysis, researchers noted a decline in semen volume with advancing age, revealing a 1.06-fold increase in the likelihood of decreased semen volumes compared to the previous year [58]. Two additional studies have documented substantial age-related declines in semen volume [11, 63]. Conversely, some authors have found no association between age and semen volume [22, 40, 49]. However, while semen volume was markedly more significant in the 18–29 age group compared to the other two cohorts, no significant disparity was detected between the 30–39 and 40–49 age groups [74]. E. Levitas et al. analyzed 6022 semen samples to investigate the correlation between age and sperm parameters. They observed a peak semen volume of 3.51 ± 1.76 ml in individuals aged ≥30–< 35 years, while the lowest volume of 2.21 ± 1.23 ml was noted in those aged ≥55 years ($P < 0.05$) [56].

## 6. Animal studies

Examining age-related alterations in semen characteristics has attracted considerable attention within the realm of reproductive biology. This exploration offers valuable insights into male animals' reproductive capabilities and longevity. Numerous animal model studies have delved into age's impact on the quality and quantity of semen, illuminating the ever-changing landscape of male fertility throughout their lifespan. For instance, it has been observed that advanced age in male dogs is associated with a decline in sperm motility and an elevated percentage of morphologically abnormal sperm [75]. The mechanism explaining age's influence on semen quality (**Figure 2**) includes reduced antioxidant defense in the seminal fluid of older animals, which could impact sperm viability [77, 78]. Impaired function of the epididymis and accessory sex glands, which may impact sperm motility [79]. Diminished germ cell counts and androgen levels; due to physiological and cellular changes, there is a decreased capacity to repair cells and tissues; aging associated genital infection and systemic disease; changes in the male reproductive anatomy, such as reduced blood flow to the testes and narrowing of the seminiferous tubules [12]. The available information suggests that older animals may undergo compromised spermatogenesis, developing morphological abnormalities in their sperm [80, 81].

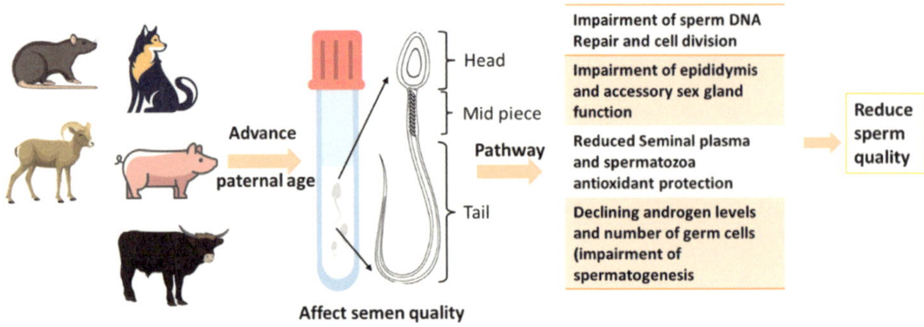


**Figure 2.**
*Possible mechanisms of sperm cell aging [76] (modified).*

A comprehensive cohort study conducted on Great Danes showed significant associations between the age of male Great Danes and specific semen parameters, namely total motility (TM), progressive motility (PM), and immotility. Their findings revealed substantial variations in these semen parameters with each passing year of age: a decline of 9.9% in TM, a reduction of 9.0% in PM, and an increase of 8.3% in immotility [82]. Notably, these observed changes in semen parameters due to aging in Great Danes were considerably more pronounced, roughly five to ten times greater, than documented in humans [83, 84]. In contrast, another study examined the effects of age on semen traits in Sahiwal bulls. Their results demonstrated that age significantly impacted all semen traits except sperm concentration ($P < 0.01$). Ejaculate volume exhibited a notable increase with the advancing age of the bulls, reaching its zenith in the age group of ≥4–<5 years before declining in the older age group of ≥5 years. A similar pattern was observed for total daily volume. The mass activity of semen also increased with the maturity of the bulls but exhibited a decline in the ≥4–<5 and ≥ 5 age groups. The highest percentage of progressive motile sperm was identified in the ≥5 age group, while the lowest was observed in the <3 and ≥ 4–<5 age groups. Sperm concentration reached its peak in the ≥3–<4 age group, with the lowest concentration seen in the <3 age group. Sperm concentration per ejaculate was higher in the ≥4–<5 age group compared to other age categories. These findings underscore the significant influence of age on semen traits, except sperm concentration [85]. Interestingly, in the case of aging male zebrafish, their offspring exhibit a higher fitness level, even though there are noticeable declines in sperm performance and mating success. This suggests that compensatory benefits associated with aging offset the decrease in fertility over time [86].

Rats and mice are mainly used as excellent animal models for exploring the mechanisms underlying male reproductive aging. The aging process in rodents seems to be associated with histological alterations in the testes and a deterioration in the quality of sperm [87, 88]. According to Tenanmura et al., in older mice, particularly those at 18 months of age, the presence of vacuoles in germ cells became noticeable, and there was a reduction in cell numbers, leading to a thinner seminiferous epithelium [87]. In ancient mice, around 33 months of age, spermatids and spermatocytes essentially vanished, indicating a severe disruption in spermatogenesis. Also, Perkening et al., [89] found that in older mice, their testes exhibited atrophy, a decrease in the number of motile sperm, and a degenerated seminiferous epithelium. These aging mice also faced challenges in mating successfully when paired with young females. Wand et al. [88] noted that total sperm production was notably decreased in older rats, specifically those at 22 and 30 months of age. We found in our studies that men ≤30 years were 1.55 times more likely to suffer from sperm progressive motility than those above 30 years, considering the demographic characteristic is skewed to more of a youthful population.

## 7. Conclusion

Current studies shed light on the influence of age on sperm quality, which is a multifaceted topic with significant implications for male reproductive health and fertility. The available literature suggests a clear association between age and various parameters of semen quality, including sperm count, motility, morphology, and DNA integrity. Semen quality is thought to offer insights into male fertility, representing a man's natural ability to reproduce, irrespective of his desire for intentional pregnancy. While research consistently indicates a decline in semen quality with advancing age, it is essential to note that individual variations exist. Not all older men experience the same level of decline. Aging affects men's reproductive organs, decreasing testis volume, testosterone level, and gonadotropin hormone and increasing oxidative stress of the sperm. Nonetheless, the collective evidence underscores the importance of considering age in assessing male fertility potential. It provides valuable insights for clinicians and researchers working in the field of reproductive medicine.

## Author details

Abdoulie Dukureh[1,2,3], Sia Florence[1,2], Balansama Marah[1,2], Peihao Wu[1,2,3], Yan Yuan[1,2], Yixuan Yan[1,2], Feng Wu[1,2], Qi Liu[1,2], Ying Li[4], Jinqi Ma[4], Feng Pan[5], Jun Ye[3], Jing Wei[3], Hongshan Ge[3*], Qiuqin Tang[6*] and Wei Wu[1,2,3*]

1 State Key Laboratory of Reproductive Medicine and Offspring Health, Center for Global Health, Nanjing Medical University, Nanjing, China

2 Key Laboratory of Modern Toxicology of Ministry of Education, School of Public Health, Nanjing Medical University, Nanjing, China

3 Taizhou Clinical Medical College, Nanjing Medical University, Taizhou, China

4 The affiliated Wuxi People's Hospital of Nanjing Medical University, Wuxi People's Hospital, Wuxi Medical Center, Nanjing Medical University, Wuxi, China

5 Department of Urology, Women's Hospital of Nanjing Medical University, Nanjing Maternity and Child Health Care Hospital, Nanjing, China

6 Department of Obstetrics, Women's Hospital of Nanjing Medical University, Nanjing Maternity and Child Health Care Hospital, Nanjing, China

*Address all correspondence to: hongshange@njmu.edu.cn, tqq19871004@126.com and wwu@njmu.edu.cn

## References

[1] Zegers-Hochschild F et al. The International Committee for Monitoring Assisted Reproductive Technology (ICMART) and the World Health Organization (WHO) revised glossary on ART terminology, 2009. Human Reproduction. 2009;**24**(11):2683-2687

[2] Kidd SA, Eskenazi B, Wyrobek AJ. Effects of male age on semen quality and fertility: A review of the literature. Fertility and Sterility. 2001;**75**(2):237-248

[3] Qiao J, Feng HL. Assisted reproductive technology in China: Compliance and non-compliance. Translational Pediatrics. 2014;**3**(2):91

[4] Boitrelle F et al. The sixth edition of the WHO manual for human semen analysis: A critical review and SWOT analysis. Life. 2021;**11**(12):1368

[5] Sharma R et al. Effects of increased paternal age on sperm quality, reproductive outcome and associated epigenetic risks to offspring. Reproductive Biology and Endocrinology. 2015;**13**:1-20

[6] Oliveira JBA et al. The effects of age on sperm quality: An evaluation of 1,500 semen samples. JBRA Assisted Reproduction. 2014;**18**(2):34

[7] Gunes S et al. Effects of aging on the male reproductive system. Journal of Assisted Reproduction and Genetics. 2016;**33**:441-454

[8] Bray I, Gunnell D, Smith GD. Advanced paternal age: How old is too old? Journal of Epidemiology & Community Health. 2006;**60**(10):851-853

[9] Einiö E, Goisis A, Myrskylä M. Is the relationship between men's age at first birth and midlife health changing? Evidence from two British cohorts. SSM - Population Health. 2019;**8**:100458

[10] Niederberger C. Re: The age of fathers in the USA is rising: An analysis of 168 867 480 births from 1972 to 2015. Journal of Urology. 2018;**199**(5):1099

[11] Verón GL et al. Impact of age, clinical conditions, and lifestyle on routine semen parameters and sperm kinematics. Fertility and Sterility. 2018;**110**(1):68-75.e4

[12] Halvaei I, Litzky J, Esfandiari N. Advanced paternal age: Effects on sperm parameters, assisted reproduction outcomes and offspring health. Reproductive Biology and Endocrinology. 2020;**18**(1):110

[13] Mahmoud A et al. Testicular volume in relation to hormonal indices of gonadal function in community-dwelling elderly men. The Journal of Clinical Endocrinology & Metabolism. 2003;**88**(1):179-184

[14] Paniagua R et al. Ultrastructure of Leydig cells in human ageing testes. Journal of Anatomy. 1986;**146**:173

[15] Levine H et al. Temporal trends in sperm count: A systematic review and meta-regression analysis. Human Reproduction Update. 2017;**23**(6):646-659

[16] Johnson SL et al. Consistent age-dependent declines in human semen quality: A systematic review and meta-analysis. Ageing Research Reviews. 2015;**19**:22-33

[17] Ford WC et al. Increasing paternal age is associated with delayed conception

in a large population of fertile couples: Evidence for declining fecundity in older men. The ALSPAC study team (Avon longitudinal study of pregnancy and childhood). Human Reproduction. 2000;**15**(8):1703-1708

[18] Neaves WB et al. Leydig cell numbers, daily sperm production, and serum gonadotropin levels in aging men. The Journal of Clinical Endocrinology and Metabolism. 1984;**59**(4):756-763

[19] Patel AS, Leong JY, Ramasamy R. Prediction of male infertility by the World Health Organization laboratory manual for assessment of semen analysis: A systematic review. Arab Journal of Urology. 2018;**16**(1):96-102

[20] Belloc S et al. How to overcome male infertility after 40: Influence of paternal age on fertility. Maturitas. 2014;**78**(1):22-29

[21] Eskenazi B et al. The association of age and semen quality in healthy men. Human Reproduction. 2003;**18**(2):447-454

[22] Stone BA et al. Age thresholds for changes in semen parameters in men. Fertility and Sterility. 2013;**100**(4):952-958

[23] Zhu Q-X et al. Turning point of age for semen quality: A population-based study in Chinese men. Fertility and Sterility. 2011;**96**(3):572-576

[24] Sloter E et al. Quantitative effects of male age on sperm motion. Human Reproduction. 2006;**21**(11):2868-2875

[25] Danis RB, Samplaski MK. Sperm morphology: History, challenges, and impact on natural and assisted fertility. Current Urology Reports. 2019;**20**:1-8

[26] Mukhopadhyay D et al. Semen quality and age-specific changes: A study between two decades on 3,729 male partners of couples with normal sperm count and attending an andrology laboratory for infertility-related problems in an Indian city. Fertility and Sterility. 2010;**93**(7):2247-2254

[27] Lemack GE, Goldstein M. Presence of sperm in the pre-vasectomy reversal semen analysis: Incidence and implications. The Journal of Urology. 1996;**155**(1):167-169

[28] Menkveld R. Clinical significance of the low normal sperm morphology value as proposed in the fifth edition of the WHO Laboratory manual for the examination and processing of human semen. Asian Journal of Andrology. 2010;**12**(1):47-58

[29] Kraemer M et al. Factors influencing human sperm kinematic measurements by the Celltrak computer-assisted sperm analysis system. Human Reproduction. 1998;**13**(3):611-619

[30] Mortimer ST, van der Horst G, Mortimer D. The future of computer-aided sperm analysis. Asian Journal of Andrology. 2015;**17**(4):545-553

[31] Khandwala YS, Baker VL, Shaw GM, Stevenson DK, Lu Y, Eisenberg ML, et al. Association of paternal age with perinatal outcomes between 2007 and 2016 in the United States: Population based cohort study. British Medical Journal. 2018;**363**:4372. DOI: 10.1136/bmj.k4372

[32] Fréour T et al. Computer-assisted sperm analysis parameters in young fertile sperm donors and relationship with age. Systems Biology in Reproductive Medicine. 2012;**58**(2):102-106

[33] Li Y et al. Trends in sperm quality by computer-assisted sperm analysis of 49,189 men during 2015-2021 in a fertility center from China. Frontiers in Endocrinology (Lausanne). 2023;**14**:1194455

[34] Shindel AW, Yan Y, Naughton CK. Does the number and size of veins ligated at left-sided microsurgical subinguinal varicocelectomy affect semen analysis outcomes? Urology. 2007;**69**(6):1176-1180

[35] Jarow JP et al. Best practice policies for male infertility. The Journal of Urology. 2002;**167**(5):2138-2144

[36] Sengupta P et al. Decline in sperm count in European men during the past 50 years. Human & Experimental Toxicology. 2018;**37**(3):247-255

[37] Hellstrom WJG et al. Semen and sperm reference ranges for men 45 years of age and older. Journal of Andrology. May/June 2006;**27**(3)

[38] Wang C et al. Evolution of the WHO "semen" processing manual from the first (1980) to the sixth edition (2021). Fertility and Sterility. 2022;**117**(2):237-245

[39] Skakkebaek NE et al. Male reproductive disorders and fertility trends: Influences of environment and genetic susceptibility. Physiological Reviews. 2016;**96**(1):55-97

[40] Li WN et al. Semen quality pattern and age threshold: A retrospective cross-sectional study of 71,623 infertile men in China, between 2011 and 2017. Reproductive Biology and Endocrinology. 2019;**17**(1):107

[41] Jensen TK et al. Poor semen quality may contribute to recent decline in fertility rates. Human Reproduction. 2002;**17**(6):1437-1440

[42] Brahem S et al. The effects of male aging on semen quality, sperm DNA fragmentation and chromosomal abnormalities in an infertile population. Journal of Assisted Reproduction and Genetics. 2011;**28**(5):425-432

[43] Collodel G et al. Influence of age on sperm characteristics evaluated by light and electron microscopies. Scientific Reports. 2021;**11**(1):4989

[44] Rumbold AR et al. Impact of male factor infertility on offspring health and development. Fertility and Sterility. 2019;**111**(6):1047-1053

[45] Khandwala YS et al. The age of fathers in the USA is rising: An analysis of 168 867 480 births from 1972 to 2015. Human Reproduction. 2017;**32**(10):2110-2116

[46] Kühnert B, Nieschlag E. Reproductive functions of the ageing male. Human Reproduction Update. 2004;**10**(4):327-339

[47] Hassan MA, Killick SR. Effect of male age on fertility: Evidence for the decline in male fertility with increasing age. Fertility and Sterility. 2003;**79**:1520-1527

[48] de La Rochebrochard E, Thonneau P. Paternal age and maternal age are risk factors for miscarriage; results of a multicentre European study. Human Reproduction. 2002;**17**(6):1649-1656

[49] Pallotti F et al. Varicocele and semen quality: A retrospective case–control study of 4230 patients from a single Centre. Journal of Endocrinological Investigation. 2018;**41**:185-192

[50] Carlsen E et al. Longitudinal changes in semen parameters in young Danish men from the Copenhagen area. Human Reproduction. 2005;**20**(4):942-949

[51] Garg J et al. Abnormal semen parameters among males in infertile couples: A cross sectional study from a tertiary care centre. International Journal of Reproduction, Contraception, Obstetrics and Gynecology. 2020;**9**(8):3398-3402

[52] Humm KC, Sakkas D. Role of increased male age in IVF and egg donation: Is sperm DNA fragmentation responsible? Fertility and Sterility. 2013;**99**(1):30-36

[53] Morris G et al. Effect of paternal age on outcomes in assisted reproductive technology cycles: Systematic review and meta-analysis. F&S Reviews. 2020;**1**(1):16-34

[54] Wyrobek AJ et al. Advancing age has differential effects on DNA damage, chromatin integrity, gene mutations, and aneuploidies in sperm. Proceedings of the National Academy of Sciences. 2006;**103**(25):9601-9606

[55] Khandwala YS et al. Association of paternal age with perinatal outcomes between 2007 and 2016 in the United States: Population based cohort study. BMJ. 2018:363

[56] Levitas E et al. Relationship between age and semen parameters in men with normal sperm concentration: Analysis of 6022 semen samples. Andrologia. 2007;**39**(2):45-50

[57] Cooper TG et al. World Health Organization reference values for human semen characteristics. Human Reproduction Update. 2010;**16**(3):231-245

[58] Pino V et al. The effects of aging on semen parameters and sperm DNA fragmentation. JBRA Assisted Reproduction. 2020;**24**(1):82-86

[59] Edition F. Examination and Processing of Human Semen. World Health [Internet]. Geneva, Switzerland: World Health Organization; 2010

[60] Auger J et al. Decline in semen quality among fertile men in Paris during the past 20 years. The New England Journal of Medicine. 1995;**332**(5):281-285

[61] Bujan L et al. Sperm morphology in fertile men and its age related variation. Andrologia. 1988;**20**(2):121-128

[62] Medicine, P.C.O.T.A.S.F.R. The clinical utility of sperm DNA integrity testing: A guideline. Fertility and Sterility. 2013;**99**(3):673-677

[63] Lai SF et al. Effect of paternal age on semen parameters and live birth rate of in-vitro fertilisation treatment: A retrospective analysis. Hong Kong Medical Journal. 2018;**24**(5):444-450

[64] Mínguez-Alarcón L et al. Hair mercury (Hg) levels, fish consumption and semen parameters among men attending a fertility center. International Journal of Hygiene and Environmental Health. 2018;**221**(2):174-182

[65] Agarwal A, Makker K, Sharma R. Clinical relevance of oxidative stress in male factor infertility: An update. American Journal of Reproductive Immunology. 2008;**59**(1):2-11

[66] Kumar S, Kumari A, Murarka S. Lifestyle factors in deteriorating male reproductive health. Indian Journal of Experimental Biology. 2009;**47**(8):615-624

[67] Evenson DP, Darzynkiewicz Z, Melamed MR. Relation of mammalian sperm chromatin heterogeneity to fertility. Science. 1980;**210**(4474):1131-1133

[68] Singh NP, Muller CH, Berger RE. Effects of age on DNA double-strand

breaks and apoptosis in human sperm. Fertility and Sterility. 2003;**80**(6):1420-1430

[69] Plastira K et al. The effects of age on DNA fragmentation, chromatin packaging and conventional semen parameters in spermatozoa of oligoasthenoteratozoospermic patients. Journal of Assisted Reproduction and Genetics. 2007;**24**(10):437-443

[70] Moskovtsev SI, Willis J, Mullen JB. Age-related decline in sperm deoxyribonucleic acid integrity in patients evaluated for male infertility. Fertility and Sterility. 2006;**85**(2):496-499

[71] Nijs M et al. Correlation between male age, WHO sperm parameters, DNA fragmentation, chromatin packaging and outcome in assisted reproduction technology. Andrologia. 2011;**43**(3):174-179

[72] Colin A et al. The effect of age on the expression of apoptosis biomarkers in human spermatozoa. Fertility and Sterility. 2010;**94**(7):2609-2614

[73] Ahadi M et al. Evaluation of the standardization in semen analysis performance according to the WHO protocols among laboratories in Tehran, Iran. Iranian Journal of Pathology. 2019;**14**(2):142

[74] Ulubay M, Ulu MB, Akdeniz E. The effect of aging on semen parameters in normozoospermic men: A cross-sectional study. International Journal of Reproductive BioMedicine. 2022;**20**(11):955

[75] Goericke-Pesch S, Failing K. Retrospective analysis of canine semen evaluations with special emphasis on the use of the hypoosmotic swelling (HOS) test and acrosomal evaluation using Spermac(®). Reproduction in Domestic Animals. 2013;**48**(2):213-217

[76] Abah KO et al. Effect of male age on semen quality in domestic animals: Potential for advanced functional and translational research? Veterinary Research Communications. 2023;**47**(3):1125-1137

[77] Pintus E, Ros-Santaella JL. Impact of oxidative stress on male reproduction in domestic and wild animals. Antioxidants. 2021;**10**(7):1154

[78] Carreira JT et al. Does sperm quality and DNA integrity differ in cryopreserved semen samples from young, adult, and aged Nellore bulls? Basic and Clinical Andrology. 2017;**27**:12

[79] Vidament M et al. Equine frozen semen: Freezability and fertility field results. Theriogenology. 1997;**48**(6):907-917

[80] Mandal DK, Kumar M, Tyagi S. Effect of age on spermiogram of Holstein Friesian × Sahiwal crossbred bulls. Animal. 2010;**4**(4):595-603

[81] Kumi-Diaka J, Nagaratnam V, Rwuaan JS. Seasonal and age-related changes in semen quality and testicular morphology of bulls in a tropical environment. The Veterinary Record. 1981;**108**(1):13-15

[82] Foutouhi A et al. Sperm parameters in the great Dane: Influence of age on semen quality. Theriogenology. 2023;**197**:267-274

[83] Fuente-Lara A et al. Effects from aging on semen quality of fresh and cryopreserved semen in Labrador retrievers. Theriogenology. 2019;**132**:164-171

[84] Hesser A et al. Semen evaluation and fertility assessment in a purebred dog breeding facility. Theriogenology. 2017;**87**:115-123

[85] Bhakat M et al. Effect of age and season on semen quality parameters in Sahiwal bulls. Tropical Animal Health and Production. 2011;**43**(6):1161-1168

[86] Johnson SL et al. Evidence that fertility trades off with early offspring fitness as males age. Proceedings of the Biological Sciences. 2018;**285**(1871):1-9

[87] Tanemura K et al. Age-related morphological changes in the testis of the BDF1 mouse. The Journal of Veterinary Medical Science. 1993;**55**(5):703-710

[88] Wang C, Leung A, Sinha-Hikim AP. Reproductive aging in the male brown-Norway rat: A model for the human. Endocrinology. 1993;**133**(6):2773-2781

[89] Parkening TA, Collins TJ, Au WW. Paternal age and its effects on reproduction in C57BL/6NNia mice. Journal of Gerontology. 1988;**43**(3):B79-B84

Chapter 2

# Spermatogenesis

*Ekementeabasi Aniebo Umoh*


## Abstract

Spermatogenesis is a complex process involving stages of spermatocytogenesis, spermatidogenesis and spermiogenesis. It is defined as the process of producing haploid sperm cells from primordial diploid germ cells in the seminiferous tubules of the testis. Hormonal role at each stage of spermatogenesis and signaling or regulatory pathways that is associated with the process has been discussed in this chapter. The factors that alters spermatogenesis which spans through hormones, medication, temperature, toxins etc., are further explained. Diagrams showing the stages of spermatogenesis and tables, which explains various alterations in genetic materials resulting in disorders of spermatogenesis, are also explained. The various stages and phases in each processes of spermatogenesis have been explained in detail. Also, chromosomal changes and cellular divisions that constitute spermatogenesis are further discussed. Finally, the role of calcium in spermatogenesis is discussed.


**Keywords:** spermatocyte, spermatogonium, spermatid, sertoli cell, sperm

## 1. Introduction

New offspring are formed following the fertilization of an ovum by sperm cells when they unite. These new offspring are often referred to as zygotes at the point of conception. Sperm cells are male reproductive cells often produced by the testis, whereas oocytes are the female gametes needed for sexual reproduction. The sperm cell is haploid in nature, containing one set of chromosomes. However, the germ cells from which the sperm cells originate are diploid in nature, containing two sets of chromosomes. The process of producing haploid sperm cells from primordial diploid germ cells in the seminiferous tubules of the testis, which is often regulated by signaling molecules, is called *spermatogenesis*. The primary essence of spermatogenesis is to produce mature male gametes and preserve the number of chromosomes in the offspring. Abnormalities in the process of spermatogenesis often result in congenital disorders such as Klinefelter syndrome, Down syndrome, and, in many cases, spontaneous abortion of the developing fetus [1–5].

## 2. Process of spermatogenesis

The process of spermatogenesis takes place at different structures of the male reproductive system. It starts from the seminiferous tubules and later progresses to the epididymis of the testis. The seminiferous tubules are tubular structures that form the testis. They consist of sertoli cells and spermatogenic cells. The sertoli cells are tall and columnar in nature, with the sole responsibility of supporting and nourishing the sperm cells, whereas the spermatogenic cells are those that eventually differentiate into the spermatozoa, or sperm cells [6]. Initially, these sperm cells are immature; however, maturation of these sperm cells occurs in the epididymis. Spermatogenesis is made up of three basic processes, namely:

1. Spermatocytogenesis

2. Spermatidogenesis

3. Spermiogenesis

Aside the process above, there exists a final stage of *spermiation* which entails the release of the matured sperm cell.

These processes cover both mitotic and meiotic divisions, each happening per given stage.

### 2.1 Spermatocytogenesis

The various stages in spermatogenesis involve the mitotic division of stem cells for the purpose of creating mature male gametocytes (sperm cells). Hence, spermatocytogenesis is usually considered the male form of gametocytogenesis, while oocytogenesis is referred to as the female form of gametocytogenesis. The stem cell of spermatogenesis is the spermatogonium, which is resident in the basal compartment of the seminiferous tubules. Spermatogonium is a cell produced at the early stage in the formation of spermatozoa. It first appears in the testis of the fetus but do not multiply significantly until after puberty. They act as stem cells in the walls of the seminiferous tubules, dividing continuously by mitosis and giving rise to spermatocytes. Spermatogonia often divides into several cell types before finally becoming the mature sperm cell. There are about one billion spermatogonia in both testicles, and they are classified into three: Type A dark spermatogonia (AD), Type A pale spermatogonia (AP), and Type B spermatogonia (B). Type AD spermatogonia are involved in maintaining the constant supply of stem cells for spermatogenesis and are not directly involved in producing sperm. They rather undergo mitotic cell division to replicate themselves. The daughter cell further goes ahead to differentiate, continuing in the process of spermatogenesis. Type AP spermatogonia often differentiates repeatedly to form Type B spermatogonia. Initially, they divide to form identical cell clones linked by cytoplasmic bridges for the purpose of synchronization of the clones. After repeated divisions have ceased, spermatogonia B is finally formed. Spermatogonia B are the cells that undergo mitotic division to form diploid primary spermatocytes, which is the ultimate aim of spermatocytogenesis (**Figure 1**). A spermatocyte is a cell produced as an intermediate stage in the formation of spermatozoa. The spermatocyte develops from spermtogonia (spermatogonia B) in the walls of the seminiferous tubules of the testis: they are either primary or secondary spermatocyte according to whether they are undergoing the first or second division of meiosis. Hence, Spermatogonia B often gives rise to primary spermatocyte, being the first

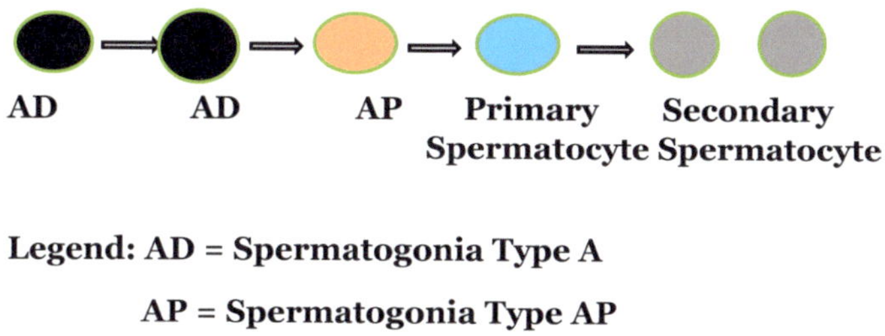


**Figure 1.**
*Cellular divisions in spermatocytogenesis.*

division of meiosis in the process of spermatogenesis. The primary spermatocyte further undergoes division to form the secondary spermatocyte [7, 8].

Type A spermatogonia bears dark, ovoid nuclei with condensed chromatin. Type AP is also referred to as Type B spermatogonia. It is pale-stained with spherical nuclei.

## 2.2 Spermatidogenesis

Spermatidogenesis is the creation of spermatid cells from secondary spermatocytes. A spermatid or spermatid cell is a small cell produced as an intermediate stage in the formation of spermatozoa. They become embedded in Sertoli cells in the testis and are often transformed into spermatozoa by the process of spermiogenesis. Previous divisions seen by cells in spermatocytogenesis were concerned with mitotic division, where a cell divides to form a singular cell at a time. However, in spermatidogenesis, a meiosis pattern of division is seen. The secondary spermatocytes enter into two rounds of division, which will give rise to four daughter cells, each having a copy of each parent's cell chromosome [9]. This makes the newly formed cell haploid in nature (**Figure 2**).

Sequel to the duration of spermatidogenesis, secondary spermatocytes can hardly be seen when cells are viewed through the microscope for histological preparations [9].

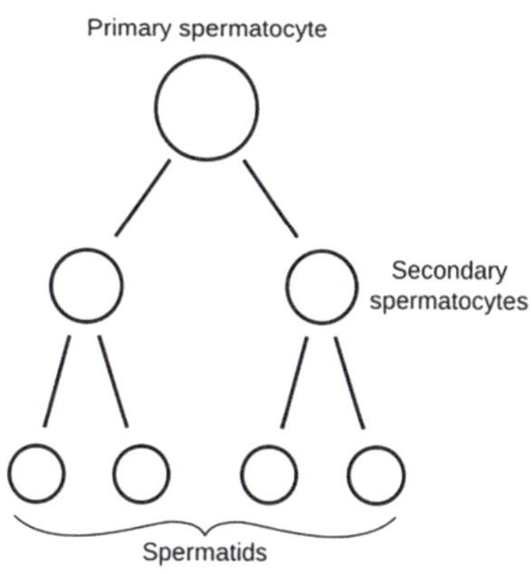


**Figure 2.**
*Stages of spermatidogenesis.*

### 2.3 Spermiogenesis

Spermiogenesis involve the development of spermatids into matured spermatozoa. Spermatozoa are matured male sex cells with a head, neck or mid-piece and a tail. It is also commonly referred to as a sperm. The tail of the sperm enables it to swim, which is important as a means for reaching and fertilizing the ovum even though muscular movement of the uterus may assist its journey from the vagina. The shape and structure of spermatid undergoes different modeling before it finally forms the matured spermatozoa. Four cellular organelles are commonly found in the spermatid at the beginning of spermiogenesis: mitochondria, centriole, nucleus and Golgi apparatus. The spermatid also appears circular or round in shape. However, after transformation, the matured spermatozoon formed becomes elongated with three outstanding structures: head, mid-piece and tail. This stage is considered the last stage of spermatogenesis [6, 10].

#### *2.3.1 Phases of spermiogenesis*

Spermiogenesis has basically four stages [6, 10, 11]: Golgi phase, cap phase, tail formation and maturation stage.

In the *Golgi stage*, the initially radially symmetrical spermatid starts developing polarity. This further leads to the formation of the head of the would-be spermatozoa at one end. The Golgi apparatus basically involves the formation of the head as it synthesizes enzymes needed to form the acrosome of the spermatozoa. Another unique structure formed in this stage is the mid-piece. The mid-piece is formed at another end of the head. A unique structure called axoneme at the midpiece is also formed following the gathering of mitochondria and the distal centriole. The Golgi stage is also characterized with spermatid DNA packaging by specific nuclear basic proteins in the nucleus. These proteins are subsequently replaced by protamines during elongation. However, the resultant tightly packed chromatin is transcriptionally inactive.

The *cap phase* is characterized with sudden gathering of the Golgi apparatus on the condensed nucleus to form the acrosomal cap.

*Tail formation* features an elongation of one of the centrioles previously found in the spermatid through the help of a temporary structure called manchette. The would-be spermatozoa usually tilt itself towards the center of the lumen, away from the epithelium.

Finally, the excess of the cytoplasm is phagocytosed by surrounding Sertoli cells in the testes. This stage is referred to the *maturation stage.* The excess cytoplasm is often referred the residual body of Regaud [6, 10, 11].

## 3. Spermiation

Spermiation is simply the process of sperm release. Here, matured spermatozoa phagocytosed by Sertoli cells are further released by the same Sertoli cells into the seminiferous tubules. This process helps to remove every cytoplasmic and organelle that is no longer needed by the mature spermatozoa. The Sertoli cells are further involved in the transport of the matured spermatozoa from the seminiferous tubules to the epididymis via the testicular fluid they often secrete and peristalsis contraction. The purpose of spermatozoa transport to the epididymis is to help them acquire motility functions. Prior to when the spermatozoa were found in the seminiferous tubules, they were not motile and hence considered sterile. It is also essential to note that the motility characteristics acquired by the matured spermatozoa cannot carry them through other aspects of the male reproductive system. Hence, their movement through the male reproductive system is achieved through muscular contractions and not the inherent motility function acquired by the spermatozoa [6].

Prior to when the sperm is traveling through the male reproductive system, the acrosome cap often prevents it from fertilizing the eggs. On entering the female reproductive tract, an enzyme called fertilization-promoting peptides (FPP) synthesized in the prostate and heparin, domicile in the female reproductive tract, takes off the acrosome coat, allowing it to bind and fertilize the egg. This process is often referred to as *capacitation* [6, 10].

## 4. Chromosomal numbers, life phases and various stages of spermatogenesis

The initial stage of spermatogenesis is characterized with diploid numbers of chromosomes. The spermatogonium cell contains 23 pairs of chromosomes summing up to 46 chromosomes. These 23 pairs of chromosomes is such that 22 of the pairs are autosomal chromosomes whereas one of the pair is the sex chromosomes. The pairs of chromosomes always feature equal contributions from both paternal and maternal parent. The sex chromosomes constitute the X and Y chromosomes. The paternal parents always have the tendency to release either an X or a Y chromosome whereas the maternal origin gives out only the X chromosome. This stage of spermatogenesis is characterized with the development of primordial germ cell or spermatogonium AD into spermatogonium and usually takes from birth to puberty age (12–14 years of age). The spermatogonium has the ability to proliferate via mitotic division inside the testis. Hence, this stage of spermatogenesis can be considered the *proliferation stage*. It is believed that a man has about seven generations of spermatogonium, i.e., the spermatogonium can divide to form itself seven times before the last one finally develops into the *primary spermatocyte*. Primary spermatocyte only undergoes growth without changes in its composition before developing into secondary spermatocyte. The chromosomal numbers of the primary spermatocyte remains the same 46, and this period constitutes the *growth stage* of spermatogenesis. The stage of growth is often followed by that of *maturation.* Each primary spermatocyte develops into a secondary spermatocyte via meiotic division with changes in the number of chromosomes. The secondary spermatocytes is characterized with haploid chromosomes (23 chromosomes) with 22 of the chromosomes being autosomal and the remaining one being a sex chromosome of either Y or X type. The next meiotic division by the secondary spermatocyte often result in the spermatid cell. The duration of spermatogenesis is such that it takes 25 days for the changes that results in the development of spermatogonium into primary spermatocyte, 9 days for primary spermatocyte to develop into secondary spermatocyte, 19 days for the development of spermatid and 21 days for the spermatid o develop into mature sperm or spermatozoa (**Figure 3**) [12, 13].

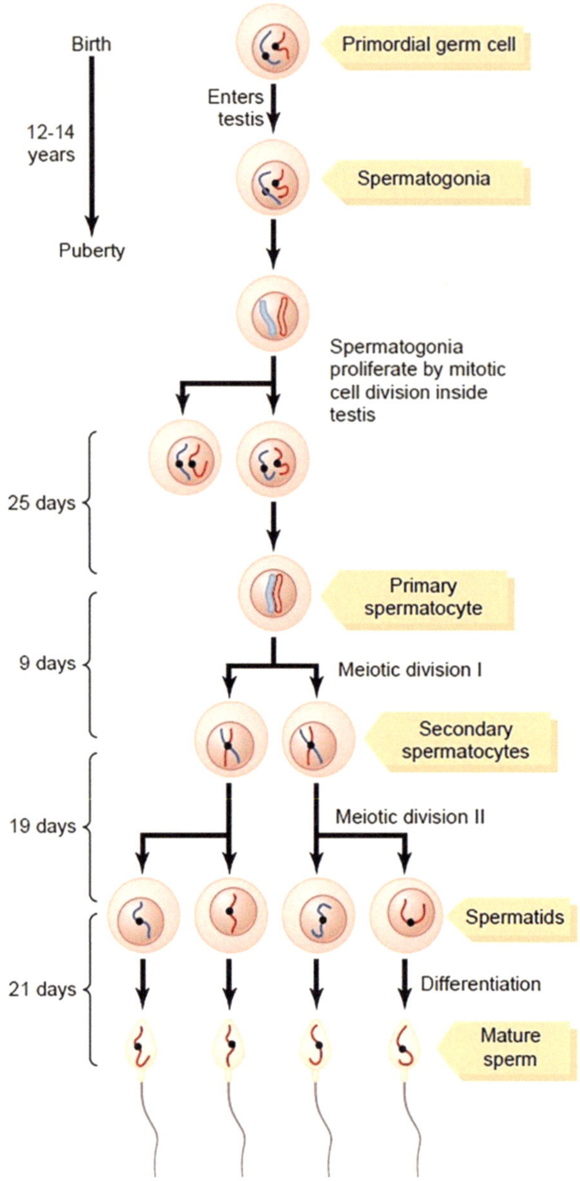


**Figure 3.**
*Cellular divisions and durations during spermatogenesis.*

## 4.1 Regulation of spermatogenesis

Spermatogenesis is regulated by the following:

1. Hormones
2. Sertoli cells
3. Temperature

4. Pathological or disease condition

5. Medications, other substances and toxins

### 4.2 Hormonal regulation of spermatogenesis

The following hormones are involve in the regulation of spermatogenesis:

1. Testosterone

2. Follicle-stimulating hormone (FSH)

3. Luteinizing hormone (LH)

4. Estrogen

5. Inhibin

6. Activin

### 4.3 Regulation of spermatogenesis by testosterone

Testosterone is involved in four critical processes during spermatogenesis namely:

1. Maintenance of blood testis barrier

2. Meiosis

3. Sertoli-spermatid adhesion and

4. Sperm release.

#### *4.3.1 Maintenance of blood testis barrier*

Testosterones are involved in regulation and coordination of tight junction which further plays out in the maintenance of the blood testis barrier integrity and allows germ cells to cross the barrier, continuing with meiotic division. Usually, there is often a transition of primary spermatocytes (preleptotene permatocyte) from the blood-testis barrier earlier formed during the late cycle of seminiferous epithelium's development with the help of Sertoli cells. This transition is aimed at forming new blood-testis barrier as the earlier ones are dissolved above the spermatocyte. During this process of transition, testosterone transports blood-testis barrier proteins of the earlier dissolved blood-testis barrier from the apical side to the basal side of the transiting germ cell. Elevated androgen receptors during this processes further buttress the fact that testosterone is involved in this process. Hence, testosterone signaling through androgen receptors is essential for remodeling and maintaining the blood-testis barrier. Certain authors has shown that testosterone signaling accelerates the kinetics of internalization of blood-testis barrier proteins from the cell surface and induce the expression of caveolin-1 and Rab11, two signaling molecules that are involved in regulating protein transcytosis and recycling, respectively. The role of testosterone in this process is also backed with their association to occludin and N-cadherin protein as these proteins together with claudin 11 and claudin 3 which are tight junction protein component of the blood-testis barrier are often found to decrease in the absence of androgen receptor [14–17].

#### *4.3.2 Meiosis*

There is little or no formation of elongated spermatids, and few germ cells can only develop to the haploid spermatid stage when there is no testosterone signaling during spermatogenesis. Since testosterone signaling is often linked to androgen receptors, elimination of androgen receptors in Sertoli cells will hinder spermatogenesis process at the stage of meiosis. Rat model experiment has shown that deprivation of testosterone has shown alterations in the expression and post-translational modification of almost 25 proteins involved in oxidative metabolism, DNA repair, RNA processing, apoptosis and meiotic division [18, 19].

#### *4.3.3 Sertoli-spermatid adhesion*

Studies from rats and mice has shown that the absence or low testosterone levels is associated with little or no elongated spermatids because round spermatids are detached from Sertoli cells prematurely. Hence, sertolispermatid adhesion could not be maintained, and germ cells are released prematurely. Adhesion proteins often affected include cadherin/cadherin and α6β1-integrin/lamininγ3 [20].

#### *4.3.4 Sperm release*

The absence of testosterone usually leads to retention and phagocytosis of matured sperm by the Sertoli cells. This effect is seen following alteration in Src protein. Activation of Src protein is essential for the release of matured sperm. Src phosphorylates β-catenin and N-cadherin, causing these proteins to diffuse away from each other, breaking their linkage and further releasing the sperm. Should there be failure in Src activation, the release of sperm is inhibited, and this is possible following the absence of testosterone [21–26].

### 4.4 Regulation of spermatogenesis by other hormones

Follicle stimulating hormones plays the initiation role of spermatogenesis. It regulates the proliferation of spermatogonia by binding with Sertoli cells and spermatogonia itself. The hormone is also involved in the formation of estrogen and androgen-binding protein from Sertoli cells [27–32].

Luteinizing hormones plays a function of secreting testosterone (a major hormone in the regulation of spermatogenesis) from the Leydig cells.

Estrogen influences four basic structures which are concerned with spermatogenesis. These include hypothalamo-pituitary-testis axis, Leydig cells, Sertoli cells, germ cells and epididymal function. Testosterone regulates the hypothalamo-pituitary axis via negative feedback mechanism. One major component of the negative feedback action of androgens on gonadotropin secretion is mediated via aromatization to estrogen. Studies have shown that administration of estradiol in humans can enhance the suppression of gonadotropin induced by testosterone-based contraceptives. Also, the presence of estrogen-binding sites in immature and adult epididymis suggest possible role of estrogen in sperm maturation and male reproduction, a point that further proof the role of estrogen in spermatogenesis. Leydig cells are often associated with the descent of testis as they produce androgens necessary for this action. Studies has also shown that exposure to estrogen can induce cryptorchidism of the male offspring by interfering with fetal hypothalamo-pituitary axis, inhibiting fetal Leydig cell androgen production and finally interfering with testicular descent. Again, Leydig cells differs in adult and fetal life. The proliferation of precursor and adult-type Leydig cells during a defined period of pubertal development is important for the establishment of the adult complement of Leydig cells. However, estrogen is often involved in inhibitory role to this process. Even neonatal estrogen exposure can interfere with Leydig cell development and proliferation during puberty. Since normal proliferation, differentiation and functional maturation of Sertoli cells is vital for spermatogenic process in fetal and adult life, inhibition of these processes by estrogen will further alter spermatogenesis and lead to infertility in males. Finally, estrogen is found to have stimulatory effect on germ cell development including spermatogonial division, germ cell viability and differentiation, acrosome biogenesis and function of spermatozoa [33–37].

Growth hormone has been linked to the regulation of spermatogenesis. General metabolic processes in the testis including proliferation of spermatogonia requires growth hormones. Evidences has shown alteration of spermatogenesis in pituitary dwarf, further buttressing the role of growth hormone in spermatogenesis [12, 13].

Activin and inhibin has complimentary effect on spermatogenesis. However, activin is found to increase the secretion of follicle stimulating hormone, accelerating spermatogenesis, and inhibin on the other side is found to regulate spermatogenesis by inhibiting the follicle stimulating hormone. Inhibin increases following an increase in the rate of spermatogenesis. This latter increase is to put the spermatogenic processes under checks as an increase in inhibin leads to a decrease in the pace of spermatogenesis [12, 13].

### 4.5 Regulation of spermatogenesis by Sertoli cells

Sertoli cells are mainly known to nourish sperm cells throughout the various stages of spermatogenesis. They are found in the convoluted part of seminiferous tubules, always appearing large and amorphous in nature. They have a distinctive dark nucleolus with their cytoplasm surrounding the germline cells that performs the nursing function. They are often stretched from the basal lamina of the seminiferous tubules to the lumen [21, 22].

Aside the nourishing of sperm cells, other functions of sertoli cell as associated to spermatogenesis include the following:

1. Phagocytic activities on residual cytoplasm during spermatogenesis [21].

2. Translocation of cells from the basal lamina to the lumen of the seminiferous tubule through conformational changes in the lateral margins of the Sertoli cells [21, 22].

3. Secretion of substances such as inhibin, activins, androgen-binding proteins and estradiol, all of which plays a significant role in spermatogenesis. Androgen-binding proteins which is otherwise known as testosterone-binding globulin, increases testosterone concentration in the seminiferous tubules to lightly stimulate spermatogenesis. Other secretory substances as associated with spermatogenesis are explained previously [22].

4. The occluding junctions of Sertoli cells are responsible for the formation of blood-testis barrier. The blood-testis barrier separates the interstitial blood compartment of the testis from the adluminal compartment of the seminiferous tubules. As a matter of fact, following the progression of spermatogonia cells from their apical portion, an essential movement that takes place during the process of spermatogenesis, there is always a need for the breaking and remodeling of the occluding junction so as to give access for the spermatogonia to cross through the blood-brain barrier and become immunologically unique. The Sertoli cells are key players in these processes as they control the entry and exit of substances (nutrient, hormones, and other chemicals) into the tubules of the testis as well as make the adluminal compartment an immune-privileged site [25, 26].

5. Sertoli cells play vital roles in the renewal of stem cells and subsequent differentiation of spermatogonia into matured germ cells. The matured germ cells further undergo several transformation during the process of spermatogenesis to become matured spermatozoa. The role of Sertoli cells further extends to sperm release (spermiation). The Sertoli cells bind continuously to the spermatogonial cells till the time of release through N-cadherin signaling molecules and galactosyltransferase (via carbohydrate residues) [22, 25, 26].

### 4.6 Regulation of spermatogenesis by temperature

Higher body temperature is known to cause infertility as spermatogenesis is altered by such temperature. Descended testis is to ensure that the temperature within the scrotom is maintained at about 2°C less than the body temperature (34–35°C) [12].

### 4.7 Regulation of spermatogenesis by disease or pathological conditions

Diseases or pathological conditions often alter spermatogenesis in a negative way. Conditions that cause impaired spermatogenesis include the following: endocrine, genetic and genitourinary disorders. Abnormalities of the hypothalamic-pituitary axis which are often related to obesity and certain thyroid gland-related disorder constitute the several endocrine disorders that alters spermatogenesis. Adrenal disorders, hyperprolactinemia, hypogonadism and hypothyroidism are often linked to impaired spermatogenesis. In all of these endocrine disorders, gonadotrophin-releasing hormone (GnRH), follicle stimulating hormone (FSH) and luteinizing hormone (LH) deficiencies are expressed. This implies why this hormonal therapy is often used as therapeutic measures in resolving certain spermatogenetic disorders. However, it is essential to know that there are no known therapeutic approaches to men when spermatogenesis is halted prior to the completion of meiosis stage of the spermatogenesis. This is always the case in many genetic disorders that lead to alteration of spermatogenesis. Genetic disorder which often impairs spermatogenesis is mostly associated to the deletion of sections of the Y chromosomes or gonadal dysgenesis. Klinefelter syndrome and cystic fibrosis are two genetic conditions linked to impaired spermatogenesis. Cystic fibrosis causes gonadal dysgenesis which subsequently results in alterations of genes linked to spermatogenesis while klinefelter syndrome results in microdeletions of sections of the Y chromosome in about 10–15 percent of men with severely impaired spermatogenesis. Cryptorchidism is one example of genitourinary disorders that impairs spermatogenesis. This may be as a result of infections such as chlamydial urethritis or gonococcal, injury, mumps orchitis, testicularatrophy

| Gene | Locus | Disorder | Gonadal manifestation | Extra-gonadal manifestation | Spermatogenesis |
|---|---|---|---|---|---|
| KAL-1 | Xp22.3 | Kallmann's syndrome | Hypotrophic testis, cryptorchidism,hypogonadism | Anosmia, renal dysplasia | Spermatiogenic arrest or quantitative reductions in germ cell proliferation |
| IC | 15q11–13 | Prader-Labhart-Willi syndrome | Hypogentalism, micropenis, hypogonadism | Stature and skeletal anomalities | Spermatogenic arrest at spermatic stage, normal fertility possible |
| DAX-1 | Xp22.2–21.3 | Congenital hypoplasia of adrenals and testis | Cryptorchidism,hypogonadism | Adrenal insufficiency | Spermatogenic arrest |
| BBS1<br>BBS2<br>BBS3<br>BBS4 | 11q13<br>16q21<br>15q22.3<br>3p12 | Laurene-Moon and Bardet-Biedel syndrome | Hypogonadism, hypogenitalism, micropenis, hypospadias | Mental retardation, obesity, retinal dystrophy | Wide range of defects in spermatogenesis, normal spermatogenesis possible |
| PIT-1 | 3p | Congenital hypopituitarism | Hypogonadism | Hypopituitarism stature anomalies | Quantitative reductions in germ cell proliferation |
| Unknown | Unknown | Isolated deficiency of FSH | Defective spermatogenesis | None | Quantitative reductions in germ cell proliferation |
| FSHR | 2p21-p16 | FSH receptor mutation | Defective spermatogenesis | None | Quantitative reductions in germ cell proliferation |
| Unknown | Unknown | Isolated deficiency of LH | Hypogionadism | None | Quantitative reductions in germ cell proliferation |
| CYP 17 | 10q24.3 | 17,20-Desmolase/17α-hydroxylase defect | Gonadal dysgenesis, cryptorchidism | Extra-gonadal effects of hypogonadism | Range of defects in spermatogenesis |
| HSD17B3 | 9q22 | 17β-Hydroxysteroid dehydrogenase defects | Gonadal dysgenesis, cryptorchidism, hypogonadism | Extra-gonadal effects of hypogonadism | Range of defects in spermatogenesis |
| SRD5A2 | 2P23 | 5α-Reductase 2 deficiency | Gonadal dysgenesis | Feminine stature | Germ cell absent, sertoli only |
| Androgen receptor (AR) | Xq11–12 | Testicular feminization, Reifenstein syndrome hypospadias, undervirilized fertile male syndrome | Feminine genitalia, abdominal testes, crrptochidism, spermatogenic lesion | Feminine phenotype, hypogonadism undervirilization, undervirilization, male phenotype | Germ cell, sertoli only, spermatid arrest at spermatid level, quantitative reduction in spermatogenesis possible |

**Table 1.**
*Gene mutation in sexual differentiation, spermatogenesis or both.*

or varicocele. Diemer and Desjardins has associated genetic causes of spermatogenesis to chromosomal aberrations. Aberrations of the chromosomes occur either as numerical or structural aberrations. In numerical aberrations, there is a missing or accessory chromosome dysfunction sequel to meiotic non-disjunction in either maternal or paternal germ cells. Often times, the cause could be linked to not just sex chromosomes but also autosomes or even both. Chromosomal aberration occurs in new born and the external genitalia of the individual affected appears normal. Assessment of the chromosomes reveals normal somatic structures, though there may be profound deviations at times. Structural aberrations on the other hand presents itself with loss or duplications of genetic information and/or translocation of genetic information from one chromosome to another without loss in a numerically normal complement of chromosomes. Microscopic inspection of karyocyte (cells that possesses a nucleus) and analysis of DNA from patient of interest is used to analyze gross structural aberration and microdeletion of gene/single base pair mutation, respectively [35–41]. **Table 1** shows the various gene mutation associated with impaired spermatogenesis [42].

### 4.8 Medications, other substances and toxin regulation of spermatogenesis

There are several substances linked to alterations in spermatogenesis. These substances include alcohol consumption in excessive amounts, anabolic steroids, androgens, antiandrogens such as bicalutamide, cyptoterone, flutamide etc., antimalarial drugs, chronic use of aspirin, excessive consumption of caffeine, cannabis, chlorambucil, cimetidine, corticosteroids, cotrimoxazole, cyclophosphamide, ethanol, estrogens, GnRH agonist which is often use for treatment of prostate cancer, ketoconazole, medroxyprogesterone, methotrexate, monoamine oxidase inhibitors, nitrofurantoin, opioids, spironolactone and sulfasalazine etc.. Also, heavy metals, pesticides, phthalamates, polychlorinated biphenyl compounds (PCBs) are certain toxins linked to alterations of spermatogenesis [43].

## 5. The role of calcium in spermatogenesis

Calcium is basically involved in the regulation of sperm motility, a function that is concerned with the spermiation process of spermatogenesis. It is also found to be involved in androgen receptor (AR) function. Mobilization of stored calcium via calcium-induced calcium release and certain agonist-induced generation of calcium mobilizing second messenger has also been linked to sperm functions especially on the aspect of capacitation of the sperm [44].

Serum calcium is maintained within narrow physiological range to normal functions of several organs as multiple cellular processes are influenced by calcium. A large fraction of calcium is protein-bound or in complex with anions such as citrate, lactate, phosphate or bicarbonate, and the free and active fraction is therefore dependent on pH and availability of binding partners [42]. Calcium and phosphate concentrations are very different in the proximal and the distal parts of the epididymis. The concentration of calcium decreases, whereas the concentration of phosphate increases. These variations in calcium and phosphate levels are believed to play a crucial role in sperm maturation and the initiation of sperm motility and in keeping the sperm quiescent during storage in the distal epididymis. The high calcium concentration in the seminal fluid may be of great importance as spermatozoa are transcriptionally silent and heavily rely on intracellular calcium as a signaling system. The concentration of total calcium in the seminal fluid is about 7·48 mM/l, and the concentration of ionized calcium is about 0·23 mM/l. Citrate and phosphate concentrations are also high in the seminal fluid, ensuring competent buffer systems and making the ionized calcium concentration lower than the corresponding serum level. Studies exploring the potential impact of the total calcium concentration in seminal fluid on sperm parameters are inconclusive – some suggest it is associated with increased motility. Magnesium, an antagonist of calcium, decreases motility in skeletal muscles and intestinal muscle supports the increased motility effect of calcium in sperm functions. Another study found an inverse relationship of calcium with sperm morphology while other research studies found no impact on sperm function at all. One study showed that low total calcium content in the seminal fluid (<5 mM/l) was associated with fewer progressive and total motile sperm and fewer morphologically normal sperm compared with men with calcium levels between 5 and 10 mM/l. Some studies has also established a linked between ionized calcium ($Ca^{2+}$) and semen quality variables. Some studies has shown positive correlation between ionized calcium and sperm motility, and others show negative correlations; while some others show no relationship. The possible link between total calcium/$Ca^{2+}$ levels and sperm motility/morphology/concentration is interesting because these semen variables are predictors of male fertility potential. However, the spermatozoa are only briefly exposed to the seminal fluid before it is mixed with female fluids, which questions a direct effect of calcium content on the fertility potential. It is also essential to note that the total calcium concentration in seminal fluid is more than 2-fold higher than the level found in serum, and the levels are not associated. Hence, there must be an active transport of calcium from serum into the seminal fluid. The calcium concentration in the different epididymal compartments (studies have only been conducted in rodents) varies largely from low to several-fold higher than the corresponding serum concentration. To maintain this steep gradient, the mechanism and proteins underlying calcium homoeostasis must be tightly regulated. Seminal fluid comprises fluid from the epididymis (about 10%), prostate (about 20%) and seminal vesicles (about 70%), which indicates that the calcium content in the ejaculate is highly dependent on secretions occurring after the transit and storage of the spermatozoa in the epididymis. At the time of ejaculation, spermatozoa escape the millimolar concentrations of citrate and phosphate in seminal fluid and encounter about 2·2 mM/l-total calcium and about 1·23 mM/l-$Ca^{2+}$ in the follicular fluid in the female reproductive tract. This influences sperm function and facilitates sperm capacitation and hyperactivation that help the sperm swim up in the vicinity of the oocyte [45–48].

Again, gene expression is silenced during spermatogenesis as histones are replaced by protamines that further condense deoxyribonucleic acid (DNA) and prevent transcription within the small spermatozoa (about 4·4 × 2·8 μM). Protein synthesis and processing are also hampered, and therefore, spermatozoa critically depend on second messenger systems to transmit extracellular signals, and they mainly rely on changes in the intracellular calcium concentration ($[Ca^{2+}]i$). An increase in $[Ca^{2+}]$ i occurs by opening $Ca^{2+}$ channels across the cell membrane or from intracellular stores – constituting a $Ca^{2+}$ signal. $[Ca^{2+}]i$ regulates capacitation, hyperactivation and the acrosome reaction. Regulation of the $[Ca^{2+}]i$ ensures the activation of spermatozoa at the appropriate time. The importance is indicated by studies showing that loss-of-function mutations in the gene coding for the main $Ca^{2+}$ channel in sperm, CatSper, lead to infertility, and spermatozoa from men in fertility treatment have lower $Ca^{2+}$ influx in response to progesterone compared with spermatozoa from healthy men. Studies have shown that men with severely impaired semen quality and men who had unsuccessful fertility treatment have significantly lower $Ca^{2+}$ influx upon stimulation with female secreted factors compared with spermatozoa from healthy men, indicating that these $Ca^{2+}$ signals are clinically relevant [45–48].

Again, certain studies has also shown the relevance of calcium and vitamin D in male fertility. In the study, it was postulated that calcium channels in male reproductive organs and spermatozoa contribute to the regulation of sperm motility and capacitation, of which both are essential for successful fertilization, which further supports a need to avoid calcium deficiency. Studies have demonstrated that vitamin D, as a regulator of calcium homoeostasis, influences calcium influx in the testis and spermatozoa. Emerging evidence suggests a potential link between vitamin D deficiency and male infertility, although further investigation is needed to establish a definitive causal relationship. Understanding the interplay between vitamin D, calcium and male reproductive health may open new avenues for improving fertility outcomes in men [45–48].

## Author details

Ekementeabasi Aniebo Umoh
Federal University Wukari, Taraba State, Nigeria

*Address all correspondence to: ekementeabasiumoh@gmail.com

## References

[1] Zhao Y, Deng S, Li C, Cao J, Wu A, Chen M, et al. The role of retinoic acid in spermatogenesis and its application in male reproduction. Cells. 2024;**13**(13):1092

[2] Sharma S, Hanukoglu A, Hanukoglu I. Localization of epithelial sodium channel (ENaC) and CFTR in the germinal epithelium of the testis, sertoli cells, and spermatozoa. Journal of Molecular Histology. 2018;**49**(2):195-208

[3] The Spermatozoön, in Gray's Anatomy. Available from: https://en.wikipedia.org/wiki/spermatozoon [Accessed: September 7, 2024]

[4] Song N, Liu J, An S, Nishino T, Hishikawa Y, Koji T. Immunohistochemical analysis of histone H3 modifications in germ cells during mouse spermatogenesis. Acta histochemica et cytochemica. 2011;**44**(4):183-190

[5] Zhang Y, Liu Z, Yun X, Batu B, Yang Z, Zhang X, et al. Transcriptome profiling of developing testes and first wave of spermatogenesis in the rat. Genes. 2023;**14**(1):229

[6] O'Donnell L, Nicholls PK, O'Bryan MK, McLachlan RI, Stanton PG. Spermiation: The process of sperm release. Spermatogenesis. 2011;**1**(1):14-35

[7] Alpatov R, Lesch BJ, Nakamoto-Kinoshita M, Blanco A, Chen S, Stützer A, et al. A chromatin-dependent role of the fragile X mental retardation protein FMRP in the DNA damage response. Cell. 2014;**157**(4):869-881

[8] Fishelson L, Gon O, Holdengreber V, Delarea Y. Comparative spermatogenesis, spermatocytogenesis, and spermatozeugmata formation in males of viviparous species of clinid fishes (Teleostei: Clinidae, Blennioidei). The Anatomical Record: Advances in Integrative Anatomy and Evolutionary Biology. 2007;**290**(3):311-323

[9] Cyranoski D. Researchers claim to have made artificial mouse sperm in a dish. Nature. 2016:10

[10] Yildirim RM, Seli E. Mitochondria as therapeutic targets in assisted reproduction. Human Reproduction. 2024:deae170

[11] Batra V, Eid N, Morgan HL, Watkins AJ. Spermatogenesis, spermiation and the human sperm. In: Mastering Clinical Embryology. Boca Raton, United States: CRC Press; 2024. pp. 82-87

[12] Gurung P, Yetiskul E, Jialal I. Physiology, Male Reproductive System [Internet]. Florida, United States: Statpearls Publishing; 2023

[13] Sembulingam K, Sembulingam P. Essentials of Medical Physiology. Delhi, India: JP Medical Ltd; 2023

[14] Pelletier RM. The blood-testis barrier: The junctional permeability, the proteins and the lipids. Progress in Histochemistry and Cytochemistry. 2011;**46**(2):49-127

[15] Wanjari UR, Gopalakrishnan AV. Blood-testis barrier: A review on regulators in maintaining cell junction integrity between sertoli cells. Cell and Tissue Research. 2024;**396**(2):157-175

[16] Yan HH, Mruk DD, Lee WM, Cheng CY. Blood-testis barrier dynamics are regulated by testosterone and

cytokines via their differential effects on the kinetics of protein endocytosis and recycling in sertoli cells. The FASEB Journal. 2008;**22**(6):1945

[17] Li XY, Zhang Y, Wang XX, Jin C, Wang YQ, Sun TC, et al. Regulation of blood–testis barrier assembly *in vivo* by germ cells. The FASEB Journal. 2018;**32**(3):1653

[18] Chang C, Chen YT, Yeh SD, Xu Q, Wang RS, Guillou F, et al. Infertility with defective spermatogenesis and hypotestosteronemia in male mice lacking the androgen receptor in sertoli cells. National Academy of Sciences of the United States of America. 2004;**101**(18):6876-6881

[19] Stanton PG, Sluka P, Foo CF, Stephens AN, Smith AI, McLachlan RI, et al. Proteomic changes in rat spermatogenesis in response to *in vivo* androgen manipulation; impact on meiotic cells. PLoS One. 2012;**7**(7):e41718

[20] Saito K, O'Donnell L, McLachlan RI, Robertson DM. Spermiation failure is a major contributor to early spermatogenic suppression caused by hormone withdrawal in adult rats. Endocrinology. 2000;**141**(8):2779-2785

[21] Lan KC, Cheng YH, Chang YC, Wei KT, Weng PL, Kang HY. Interaction between chromodomain Y-like protein and androgen receptor signaling in sertoli cells accounts for spermatogenesis. Cells. 2024;**13**(10):851

[22] Kopera IA, Bilinska B, Cheng CY, Mruk DD. Sertoli–germ cell junctions in the testis: A review of recent data. Philosophical Transactions of the Royal Society B: Biological Sciences. 2010;**365**(1546):1593-1605

[23] Wong CH, Xia W, Lee NP, Mruk DD, Lee WM, Cheng CY. Regulation of ectoplasmic specialization dynamics in the seminiferous epithelium by focal adhesion-associated proteins in testosterone-suppressed rat testes. Endocrinology. 2005;**146**(3):1192-1204

[24] Zhang J, Mruk DD, Cheng CY. Myotubularin phosphoinositide phosphatases, protein phosphatases, and kinases: Their roles in junction dynamics and spermatogenesis. Journal of Cellular Physiology. 2005;**204**(2):470-483

[25] Zhang J, Wong CH, Xia W, Mruk DD, Lee NP, Lee WM, et al. Regulation of sertoli-germ cell adherens junction dynamics via changes in protein-protein interactions of the N-cadherin-β-catenin protein complex which are possibly mediated by c-Src and myotubularin-related protein 2: An *in vivo* study using an androgen suppression model. Endocrinology. 2005;**146**(3):1268-1284

[26] Wang RS, Yeh S, Chen LM, Lin HY, Zhang C, Ni J, et al. Androgen receptor in sertoli cell is essential for germ cell nursery and junctional complex formation in mouse testes. Endocrinology. 2006;**147**(12):5624-5633

[27] Roura S, Miravet S, Piedra J, de Herreros AG, Dunach M. Regulation of E-cadherin/catenin association by tyrosine phosphorylation. Journal of Biological Chemistry. 1999;**274**(51):36734-36740

[28] Xia W, Cheng CY. TGF-β3 regulates anchoring junction dynamics in the seminiferous epithelium of the rat testis via the Ras/ERK signaling pathway: An *in vivo* study. Developmental Biology. 2005;**280**(2):321-343

[29] Kinch MS, Clark GJ, Der CJ, Burridge K. Tyrosine phosphorylation regulates the adhesions of ras-transformed breast epithelia. The Journal of Cell Biology. 1995;**130**(2):461-471

[30] O'Donnell L, Pratis K, Wagenfeld A, Gottwald U, Müller J, Leder G, et al. Transcriptional profiling of the hormone-responsive stages of spermatogenesis reveals cell-, stage-, and hormone-specific events. Endocrinology. 2009;**150**(11):5074-5084

[31] Shang Y, Myers M, Brown M. Formation of the androgen receptor transcription complex. Molecular Cell. 2002;**9**(3):601-610

[32] Abney TO. The potential roles of estrogens in regulating Leydig cell development and function: A review. Steroids. 1999;**64**(9):610-617

[33] Tsubota T, Howell-Skalla L, Nitta H, Osawa Y, Mason JI, Meiers PG, et al. Seasonal changes in spermatogenesis and testicular steroidogenesis in the male black bear *Ursus americanus*. Reproduction. 1997;**109**(1):21-27

[34] Kwon S, Hess RA, Bunick D, Nitta H, Janulis L, Osawa Y, et al. Rooster testicular germ cells and epididymal sperm contain P450 aromatase. Biology of Reproduction. 1995;**53**(6):1259-1264

[35] Congy J, Rahib D, Leroy C, Bouyer J, de La Rochebrochard E. Contraceptive use measured in a national population–based approach: Cross-sectional study of administrative versus survey data. JMIR Public Health and Surveillance. 2024;**10**:e45030

[36] Corona G, Rastrelli G, Sparano C, Vignozzi L, Sforza A, Maggi M. Pharmacological management of testosterone deficiency in men current advances and future directions. Expert Review of Clinical Pharmacology. 2024

[37] Bagatell CJ, Dahl KD, Bremner WJ. The direct pituitary effect of testosterone to inhibit gonadotropin secretion in men is partially mediated by aromatization to estradiol. Journal of Andrology. 1994;**15**(1):15-21

[38] Hayes FJ, DeCruz S, Seminara SB, Boepple PA, Crowley WF Jr. Differential regulation of gonadotropin secretion by testosterone in the human male: Absence of a negative feedback effect of testosterone on follicle-stimulating hormone secretion. The Journal of Clinical Endocrinology & Metabolism. 2001;**86**(1):53-58

[39] Hayes FJ, Seminara SB, DeCruz S, Boepple PA, Crowley WF Jr. Aromatase inhibition in the human male reveals a hypothalamic site of estrogen feedback. The Journal of Clinical Endocrinology & Metabolism. 2000;**85**(9):3027-3035

[40] Xiong X, Wang A, Liu G, Liu H, Wang C, Xia T, et al. Effects of p, p′-dichlorodiphenyldichloroethyl ene on the expressions of transferrin and androgen-binding protein in rat sertoli cells. Environmental Research. 2006;**101**(3):334-339

[41] Skinner MK, Griswold MD. Sertoli cells synthesize and secrete a ceruloplasmin-like protein. Biology of Reproduction. 1983;**28**(5):1225-1229

[42] Diemer T, Desjardins C. Developmental and genetic disorders in spermatogenesis. Human Reproduction Update. 1999;**5**(2):120-140

[43] Rebar RW. Sperm Disorder. Available from: https://www.msdmanuals.com/professional/gynecology-and-obstetrics/infertility-and-recurrent-pregnancy-loss/sperm-disorders [Accessed: July 28, 2024]

[44] Correia J, Michelangeli F, Publicover S. Regulation and roles of $Ca^{2+}$ stores in human sperm. Reproduction. 2015;**150**(2):R65-R76

[45] Hamroun A, Pekar JD, Lionet A, Ghulam A, Maboudou P, Mercier A, et al. Ionized calcium: Analytical challenges and clinical relevance. Journal of Laboratory and Precision Medicine. 2020:5

[46] Blomberg Jensen M, Bjerrum PJ, Jessen TE, Nielsen JE, Joensen UN, Olesen IA, et al. Vitamin D is positively associated with sperm motility and increases intracellular calcium in human spermatozoa. Human Reproduction. 2011;**26**(6):1307-1317

[47] Umoh EA, Obembe AO, Ikpi DE, Eniang-Esien OE, Asuquo JO, Effiom-Ekaha OO. Effect of chronic administration of magnesium supplement (magnesium glycinate) on male albino wistar rats' intestinal (ileum) motility, body weight changes, food and water intake. Heliyon. 2023;**9**(8)

[48] Yahyavi SK, Boisen IM, Cui Z, Jorsal MJ, Kooij I, Holt R, et al. Calcium and vitamin D homoeostasis in male fertility. Proceedings of the Nutrition Society. 2024;**83**(2):95-108

Chapter 3

# Natural Sperm Selection: Perspectives for More Successful Outcomes in ICSI

*Mahin Izadi, Serajoddin Vahidi, Mohammad Ebrahim Rezvani and Behrouz Aflatoonian*

**Abstract**

Natural sperm selection in the female reproductive tract involves complicated processes that result in the most competent sperm reaching the fertilization site. This selection is based on various sperm characteristics, including motility, viability, and DNA integrity. Assisted reproductive technologies (ARTs) often bypass these natural selection barriers, leading to concerns about treatment success and offspring health. Nowadays, many researchers are using these biomimetic methods of sperm selection that mimic the selection process occurring in the female reproductive tract. These methods apply microfluidic devices that separate sperm on the basis of guidance mechanisms, such as rheotaxis, chemotaxis, and thermotaxis, and the techniques have also been developed to separate sperm potential biomarkers involved in the sperm binding to the egg envelopes, such as hyaluronic acid and zona pellucida. Conclusively, application of these biomimetic methods could enhance the ART outcomes.

**Keywords:** rheotaxis, chemotaxis, thermotaxis, hyaluronic acid, zona pellucida

## 1. Introduction

The male factor infertility accounts for 50% of the total cases of human infertility, of which the well-established causes of male infertility are genetic and anatomical defects [1], expressing a considerable burden on human healthcare systems [2]. In the bygone years, medical treatment decisions relied on conventional methods for semen analysis to evaluate sperm concentration, motility, and morphology. Although the analysis of semen is important because it shows the proper function in sperm production by the testicles, the secretory function of all accessory glands, and the patency of the reproductive tract [3], these parameters become less credible indicators of male fertility potential evaluation. Precise analysis of sperm function is essential for accurate diagnosis and an appropriate treatment plan for male infertility, but a comprehensive review of semen analysis is beyond the scope of this chapter. Along with the initial reports on intracytoplasmic sperm injection (ICSI), although it seems that ICSI has become a powerful tool in the treatment of male factor infertility cases, there are still many cases of low or absent fertilization rates [4]. This actually indicates that other factors may be involved that cannot be detected by the standard magnification used in conventional ICSI. Accordingly, there are traditional and advanced approaches to the selection of appropriate sperm, with the aim of improving fertilization rate, embryo quality, and pregnancy outcomes. The use of animal models in relation to the natural selection of human sperm, due to the diversity of mating strategies in animals and differences in reproductive system and function, makes comparisons very difficult, and indeed, more details on human experiments are needed. Therefore, it is necessary to search for better methods to mimic sperm selection that occurs naturally in the female reproductive system to select the most competent sperm.

## 2. Natural sperm selection

### 2.1 Sperm upward movement and dynamics

When sperms pass through the female reproductive tract and undergo various interactions in multiple ways that facilitate their migration toward the egg, a number game process is used to reach the necessary numbers required in the fertilization area, and at the same time, proper sperm selection is done to increase the chance of fertilization [5]. Considering sperms can survive a relatively long time (≈120 hours), the cells must keep their fertility power constant, despite the limited metabolic resources when moving against multiple obstacles and opposition in the reproductive tract [6].

### 2.2 Sperm voyage and propagation in the vagina, cervix, uterus, and uterotubal junction

In humans, semen deposition takes place near the anterior vagina, adjacent to the cervical entrance. Its propagation faces vaginal pH, immune responses, and several difficulties [7] that cause considerable sperm loss and low-level sperm retention [8]. It has been found that in 94% of sexual intercourses, sperm flowback was performed within 30 minutes; on the other hand, 1.5–3 minutes after the deposition of the semen, sperms were found in the endocervix [9], which appears to show that sperms have escaped the significant cellular immune response in the vagina to the cervix [10]. The sperm-rich fraction of semen unifies into a gelatinous mass in a minute after sexual intercourse, which can act as a cervical plug to keep the sperm-rich fraction from flowing back, the vaginal environment, and rejection [11]. Within a short time after the enzymatic degradation of semen coagulum, sperm can rapidly enter and propagate in the cervical mucus, which has the highest antibacterial function; the place can be optimal for sperm transport at the midcycle of menstruation due to the hydrated mucus [12, 13]. The cervical mucus acts as an active filter, which allows the sperm with progressive motility to pass this barrier efficiently and filter out the poor motility and abnormal morphology of the sperm [14]. Highly motile sperms are found in the human cervix up to 5 days after insemination and appear to be trapped in the cervical crypts [15]. Sperms enter the uterus after passing the cervical mucus and rapidly progress to this site through peristaltic contractions [16] and pro-ovarian contractions of the myometrium [17]. There are a low number of spermatozoa in the uterus compared with the number of spermatozoa inseminated in the vagina [17]. It would be informative to investigate what we can learn from *in vivo* natural sperm selection to improve success rates of assisted reproductive technologies (ARTs) [18]. The human uterotubal junction is narrow, has mucosal folds, and is filled with viscous mucus, whose viscosity is dependent on the plasma level of estrogen. This viscous mucus flows against the direction of the sperm movement to filter out the poor quality sperm [19]. It has been demonstrated that spermatozoa display intense interaction with epithelial cells of the fallopian tube, and this interaction can cause the selection and transport of normal sperms in the human uterine tube [20]; in addition, this phenomenon may be a description of the fact that normal morphology and motility are not sufficient for sperm selection and transport in the human uterine tube and that sperm surface proteins are also required for fertilization [21].

### 2.3 Natural sperm selection in assisted reproduction

Despite several decades of research, there are many questions still remaining to be clarified about the sperm population selected in the oviduct: first, what makes the sperms different from others and special to reach the fertilization site, and second, whether these special sperms or sperms selected by a similar natural mechanism can increase the success rate of ART? Whether some natural sperm selection mechanisms that occur *in vivo* can be used to improve ART laboratory's quality? Understanding these mechanisms may give insight into the development of sperm quality assessment beyond the World Health Organization (WHO) guidelines.

The main components of a sperm cell that are involved in fertilization include the head containing the genomic material, the midpiece containing the mitochondria, and the flagellum that generates its movement. Additionally, sperms have the special mechanisms for oocyte recognition, fusion, and various intracellular factors that are effective in the process of fertilization and embryonic development [22]. The above-mentioned actions are related to different kinds of molecules that are physiologically important, and their assessment will have a place in the analysis of semen and sperm selection in the future [23].

There are different active and passive obstacles in the female reproductive tract, including vaginal pH, cervical mucus [24], and peristaltic contractions in the uterus [25] that contribute to eliminating the less functional spermatozoa. It is well established that sperms move toward certain guides during their voyage, for example, rheotaxis, chemotaxis, and thermotaxis [26]. After crossing the main barriers and reaching the fertilization site in the oviductal ampulla and oocyte, the selection of sperm does not end there but must pass through other checkpoints around the oocyte, including hyaluronic acid (HA) matrix [27] and the zona pellucida (ZP) [27–29].

Considering that ICSI is a practical reproduction technology that is used for the treatment of about half of the couples with male factor infertility, the natural sperm selection barriers mentioned above can be bypassed to achieve fertilization [30]. Therefore, it is necessary to design appropriate strategies to help in selecting functionally competent sperm.

## 3. Current standard sperm selection/preparation methods in assisted reproduction

### 3.1 Swim-up and density gradient centrifugation (DGC)

The swim-up (SU) techniques, as a migration approach, seem to somewhat mimic the natural process of sperm migration through the cervical mucus, and sperm separation occurs based on motility parameters. But this is far from the sperm motility aspect and migration that occur *in vivo*. In the SU method, sperms swim out of the liquefied semen placed into a centrifuge tube bottom that is overlaid with a sperm medium. This method can be applied to separate sperms with normal motility that are collected in the upper-layer culture medium [31].

In DGC techniques, as a sedimentation approach, semen samples are placed on the density gradient layer(s), which contain silane-coated colloidal silica, to separate spermatozoa based on their density. Even so, the use of sperm with DNA damage after sperm separation during ART may result in a suboptimal pregnancy outcome. To determine the advantages and disadvantages of new and advanced methods of sperm selection, comparative studies against the current methods, which are considered the gold standard for sperm separation, should be investigated [32].

## 4. Novel *in vitro* model for natural sperm selection

### 4.1 Rheotaxis

Rheotaxis, as a long-range sperm guidance mechanism and a passive process, occurs during the sperm's journey from the vagina to the oocyte. Sperms swim with or against fluid flow to create a chance for fertilization [33]. The ability of sperms to swim against the current is known as positive rheotaxis. According to recent research, the percentage of positively rheotactic sperm (PR%) in humans is associated with fertility, with fertile males having a greater PR%; therefore, this phenomenon can be used as a predictive marker of male fertility [34]. To isolate a cohort of sperm with high fertilization potential, microfluidic systems have been developed to mimic the movements of sperm in the female reproductive tract, the cervix canal, the lumen of the uterine tubes, and the complex epithelium of the uterine tubes. A few of these systems facilitate sperm selection over various flow gradients and biophysical forces by generating a real fluid environment.

While some new findings propose that sperm rheotaxis in humans is a passive physical process, there is no active signal transduction during human sperm rheotaxis [35]. Others postulate that it might entail adaptive fluid flow and active sense [36]. Current advances in emerging microfluidic technologies have been developed to study and exploit this phenomenon for sperm selection, offering potential improvements in ART [37]. Recent studies have demonstrated that the swimming behavior of sperm, such as rheotaxis, can be used to separate sperm with high DNA integrity, normal motility, morphology, and viability [18, 38, 39]. Based on these results, rheotaxis-based sperm selection techniques may enhance the effectiveness of ART by imitating the natural selection mechanisms occurring in the female reproductive tract.

### 4.2 Thermotaxis

The ability of sperm to detect and swim toward the warmer fertilization site along a temperature gradient is called sperm thermotaxis (this temperature difference is maintained for at least 10 hours after ovulation) [40]. It seems to be a long-range guidance mechanism that can be complementary to chemotaxis to guide the sperm toward the oocyte [41]. Although the molecular mechanisms of sperm thermotaxis remain unclear, new findings have provided insight into possible thermosensors [42]. It has been shown recently that mammalian sperms possess a complex thermal detection system, utilizing opsins like rhodopsin and melanopsin to sense temperature changes and activating different signaling pathways for thermotaxis [43]. Michael Eisenbach and colleagues recently showed that different opsins are involved in human sperm thermotaxis via two signaling pathways—the phospholipase C and the cyclic-nucleotide pathways [44]. Integrated microfluidic devices have been developed to evaluate sperm responses to thermotaxis, providing insights into sperm behavior under physiological conditions [45]. Thermotaxis is a natural mechanism that guides competent sperms through the female genital tract, therefore, imitating this method as a novel technique can cause improvement in the ART outcomes [46].

### 4.3 Chemotaxis

Egg envelope-originated factors guide the sperm toward the oocyte; this behavior is called chemotaxis [47], which occurs in close proximity to the oocyte [41], a short-range mechanism that has synergistic effects with rheotaxis on guiding the sperm toward female gametes by chemoattractants. There is evidence showing the involvement of intracellular calcium concentration ($[Ca^{2+}]_i$) [48] and chemotactic signaling cascade activation in sperm chemotaxis [49], which controls flagellar movement and sperm swimming [50]. It seems that progesterone acts as a chemoattractant for human sperm and initiates a series of signaling pathways [51]. Defects or inhibitions in this signaling pathway can cause infertility [47]. Studies have shown a role for chemotaxis in sperm selection in a study proposing that it selectively separates capacitated sperm for fertilization [52]. Also, a study established the potential of microfluidic devices for sperm chemotaxis in the selection of high-quality sperm [53]. Therefore, sperm chemotaxis may be used as a diagnostic tool for sperm quality and male infertility, and it may also be used as a natural sperm selection method in ART.

### 4.4 Hyaluronic acid (HA) binding

Hyaluronic acid (HA) serves as a key component of the cumulus oophorus extracellular matrix and plays a crucial role in various reproductive processes, including folliculogenesis, oocyte maturation, and fertilization. It has been found that mature spermatozoa are able to bind and penetrate into this matrix [54]. The hyaluronic acid-binding assay (HBA), a commercial diagnostic kit, was first introduced in the early 2000s to measure the capability of mature sperm to bind to hyaluronic acid (HA, also known as hyaluronan). This principle suggests that spermatozoa that express HA-binding sites that attach to HA-coated surfaces from their head region are those that have higher capacities to bind to the zona pellucida, higher fertilization abilities, advanced chromatin maturation, lower DNA fragmentation, lower aneuploidy rate, and superior morphology [55]. The results of studies on HA-based sperm selection for

ICSI are highly contradictory. Some studies have found that HA-binding sperm selection can increase implantation rates and high embryo quality [56, 57] can also reduce the frequency of chromosomal abnormalities in selected sperm [58]. Other studies, however, have found no significant changes in DNA integrity between HA-binding sperm and conventional sperm selection [59]. Numerous clinical studies have focused on the topic of physiological selection of spermatozoa for ICSI (P-ICSI), as a HA-based sperm selection method, which attracts significant attention. P-ICSI-selected sperm and traditional ICSI groups have been compared in cases of recurrent pregnancy loss [60], high DNA fragmentation [61], and high teratozoospermia [62], and contradictory findings have been documented. To conclusively prove that HA-based sperm selection as a physiological indicator improves ART results, more extensive research is required.

### 4.5 Zona pellucida (ZP) binding

The human zona pellucida, composed of four glycoproteins, includes zona pellucida 1 (ZP1), zona pellucida 2 (ZP2), zona pellucida 3 (ZP3), and zona pellucida 4 (ZP4) [63]. The ZP1, ZP3, and ZP4 bind to capacitated sperm, while ZP2 binds to acrosome-reacted sperm [64]. Previous research has shown that ZP-bound spermatozoa have superior morphology, DNA integrity, and chromatin structure than unbound sperm, indicating that ZP proteins are crucial for the selection of competent sperm in humans [65]. A small fraction of motile spermatozoa that display higher levels of ZP-binding proteins like heat shock 70 kDa protein 2 (HSPA2) and sperm acrosome associated 3 (SPACA3) tend to selectively interact with the ZP [66]. Spermatozoa with acrosomal abnormalities are less likely to be selected for than normal or slightly abnormal spermatozoa [65]. Using ZP as a last sperm selection filter for entering the oocyte in the female reproductive system for *in vitro* natural sperm selection methods in ART has shown promising results [29, 67]. According to a recent study, using sperm bound to immobilized and isolated ZP proteins from oocytes with a germinal vesicle (GV) can reduce the risk of miscarriage and increase the chances of pregnancy [68]. Other research shows that using sperm that is bound to ZP resulted in high-quality embryos [67, 69]. These results indicate that ZP-mediated sperm selection is a key step in human fertilization, with potential applications in assisted reproduction techniques to increase fertilization rates and decrease genetic risks (**Figure 1**).

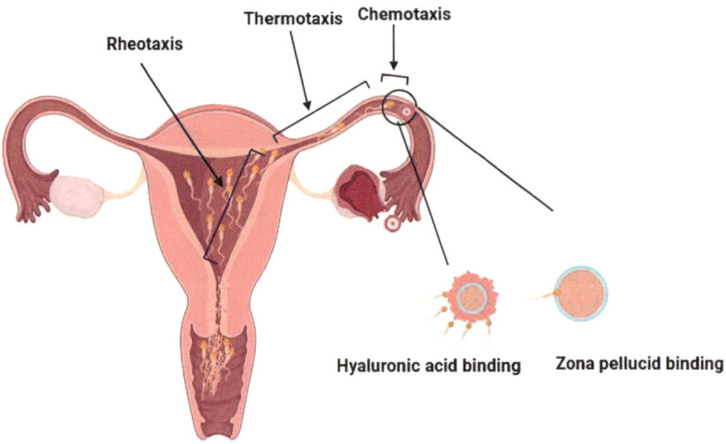


**Figure 1.**
*The mechanisms of sperm guidance and the process of natural sperm selection in the female reproductive tract. The scheme, not depicted to scale, is based on the human tract.*

## 5. Summary and future aspects

*In vitro* sperm selection techniques are used in assisted reproductive techniques (ARTs), such as ICSI or *in vitro* fertilization (IVF) insemination, to maximize the likelihood that an effective spermatozoon will be involved in fertilization. Understanding natural sperm selection mechanisms in assisted reproduction can help improve the success rate of ART and improve sperm quality assessment beyond World Health Organization (WHO) guidelines.

Several obstacles in the female reproductive tract, such as the vaginal pH, cervical mucus, and peristaltic contractions, contribute to the elimination of less functional spermatozoa. Sperms move toward the guides like rheotaxis, thermotaxis, and chemotaxis during their journey. In assisted reproduction technology, such as ICSI, natural sperm selection barriers can be bypassed to achieve fertilization. Sperm rheotaxis is a passive process and a long-range guidance mechanism where sperm swims with or against fluid flow to create a chance for fertilization. Sperm thermotaxis is also a long-range guidance mechanism that guides sperm toward the warmer fertilization site along a temperature gradient. It is a complementary mechanism to chemotaxis, which occurs in close proximity to the oocyte. Sperm chemotaxis, a short-range mechanism, has synergistic effects with rheotaxis, guiding sperm toward the female gamete by chemoattractants. Studies have shown that imitating these *in vivo* methods as novel techniques appears to be effective in selecting functional sperm for assisted reproduction techniques. The HA binding is a key component of the cumulus oophorus extracellular matrix and plays a crucial role in reproductive processes. The HBA measures revealed that the spermatozoa with HA-binding sites have higher capacities to bind to the zona pellucida, higher fertilization abilities, advanced chromatin maturation, lower DNA fragmentation, a lower aneuploidy rate, and superior morphology. However, the results of HA-based sperm selection for ICSI are highly contradictory and more extensive researches are needed to conclusively prove that HA-based sperm selection can improve ART results. ZP binding is crucial for the selection of competent sperm in humans, and using ZP as a last sperm selection filter for entering the oocyte in the female reproductive system for *in vitro* natural sperm selection methods in ART has shown promising results.

In sum, the innovative approaches like physiological ICSI and utilizing *in vivo* properties like rheotaxis, thermotaxis, and chemotaxis are paving the way in the future for precision male infertility diagnosis and treatment, with current researches aiming to confirm their advantages, particularly in reducing miscarriage rates and potentially enhancing the high-quality embryo, live birth rates, and long-term health of offspring.

## Author details

Mahin Izadi[1,2]*, Serajoddin Vahidi[1,2], Mohammad Ebrahim Rezvani[3]
and Behrouz Aflatoonian[4]

1 Research and Clinical Center for Infertility, Yazd Reproductive Sciences Institute, Shahid Sadoughi University of Medical Sciences, Yazd, Iran

2 Andrology Research Center, Yazd Reproductive Sciences Institute, Shahid Sadoughi University of Medical Sciences, Yazd, Iran

3 Department of Physiology, School of Medicine, Shahid Sadoughi University of Medical Sciences and Health Services, Yazd, Iran

4 Stem Cell Biology Research Center, Yazd Reproductive Sciences Institute, Shahid Sadoughi University of Medical Sciences, Yazd, Iran

*Address all correspondence to: mizadi890112@gmail.com

## References

[1] Vashisht A, Gahlay G. Using miRNAs as diagnostic biomarkers for male infertility: Opportunities and challenges. Molecular Human Reproduction. 2020;**26**(4):199-214

[2] Van Hoogenhuijze N, van Eekelen R, Mol F, Schipper I, Groenewoud E, Traas M, et al. Economic evaluation of endometrial scratching before the second IVF/ICSI treatment: A cost-effectiveness analysis of a randomized controlled trial (SCRaTCH trial). Human Reproduction. 2022;**37**(2):254-263

[3] Centola GM. Semen assessment. Urologic Clinics. 2014;**41**(1):163-167

[4] Sakkas D, Katz-Jaffe MG, Sueldo CE, Sueldo CE. Assessment and selection of human sperm for ART. In: Gamete and Embryo Selection: Genomics, Metabolomics and Morphological Assessment. New York, Heidelberg, Dordrecht, London. Springer; 2014. pp. 29-45

[5] Suarez SS. Mammalian sperm interactions with the female reproductive tract. Cell and Tissue Research. 2016;**363**:185-194

[6] Mortimer D, Barratt CL, Björndahl L, De Jager C, Jequier AM, Muller CH. What should it take to describe a substance or product as 'sperm-safe'. Human Reproduction Update. 2013;**19**(suppl_1):i1-i45

[7] Boskey E, Cone R, Whaley K, Moench T. Origins of vaginal acidity: High D/L lactate ratio is consistent with bacteria being the primary source. Human Reproduction. 2001;**16**(9):1809-1813

[8] Baker RR, Bellis MA. Human sperm competition: Ejaculate manipulation by females and a function for the female orgasm. Animal Behaviour. 1993;**46**(5):887-909

[9] Sobrero AJ, MacLeod J. The immediate postcoital test. Fertility and Sterility. 1962;**13**(2):184-189

[10] Sharkey DJ, Macpherson AM, Tremellen KP, Mottershead DG, Gilchrist RB, Robertson SA. TGF-β mediates proinflammatory seminal fluid signaling in human cervical epithelial cells. The Journal of Immunology. 2012;**189**(2):1024-1035

[11] Harper M. Gamete and zygote transport. In: The Physiology of Reproduction. Vol. 1. Raven Press; 1994. pp. 123-188

[12] Katz D, Slade D, Nakajima S. Analysis of pre-ovulatory changes in cervical mucus hydration and sperm penetrability. Advances in Contraception. 1997;**13**:143-151

[13] Katz DF, Drobnis EZ, Overstreet JW. Factors regulating mammalian sperm migration through the female reproductive tract and oocyte vestments. Gamete Research. 1989;**22**(4):443-469

[14] Mortimer D, Leslie E, Kelly R, Templeton A. Morphological selection of human spermatozoa in vivo and in vitro. Reproduction. 1982;**64**(2):391-399

[15] Gould JE, Overstreet JW, Hanson FW. Assessment of human sperm function after recovery from the female reproductive tract. Biology of Reproduction. 1984;**31**(5):888-894

[16] Kunz G, Beil D, Deininger H, Wildt L, Leyendecker G. The dynamics of rapid sperm transport through the female genital tract: Evidence from

vaginal sonography of uterine peristalsis and hysterosalpingoscintigraphy. Human Reproduction. 1996;**11**(3):627-632

[17] Lyons EA, Taylor PJ, Zheng XH, Ballard G, Levi CS, Kredentser JV. Characterization of subendometrial myometrial contractions throughout the menstrual cycle in normal fertile women. Fertility and Sterility. 1991;**55**(4):771-774

[18] Pardiñas ML, Martin A, Ortega-Jaén D, De los Santos JM, Viloria T, Gamiz P, et al. Sperm DNA fragmentation and microfluidics: A new era in human sperm selection. Medicina Reproductiva y Embriología Clínica. 2022;**9**(3):100121

[19] Mortimer D, Björndahl L, Barratt CL, Castilla JA, Menkveld R, Kvist U, et al. A Practical Guide to Basic Laboratory Andrology. United States: Elsevier Inc.; 2022

[20] Pacey A, Hill C, Scudamore I, Warren M, Barratt C, Cooke I. Andrology: The interaction in vitro of human spermatozoa with epithelial cells from the human uterine (Fallopian) tube. Human Reproduction. 1995;**10**(2):360-366

[21] Nakanishi T, Isotani A, Yamaguchi R, Ikawa M, Baba T, Suarez SS, et al. Selective passage through the uterotubal junction of sperm from a mixed population produced by chimeras of calmegin-knockout and wild-type male mice. Biology of Reproduction. 2004;**71**(3):959-965

[22] Krawetz SA. Paternal contribution: New insights and future challenges. Nature Reviews. Genetics. 2005;**6**(8):633-642

[23] Barratt CL, Mansell S, Beaton C, Tardif S, Oxenham SK. Diagnostic tools in male infertility—The question of sperm dysfunction. Asian Journal of Andrology. 2011;**13**(1):53

[24] Holt WV, Fazeli A. The oviduct as a complex mediator of mammalian sperm function and selection. Molecular Reproduction and Development. 2010;**77**(11):934-943

[25] Kunz G, Beil D, Huppert P, Leyendecker G. Oxytocin—A stimulator of directed sperm transport in humans. Reproductive Biomedicine Online. 2007;**14**(1):32-39

[26] Suarez S, Wu M. Microfluidic devices for the study of sperm migration. MHR: Basic Science of Reproductive Medicine. 2017;**23**(4):227-234

[27] Huszar G, Jakab A, Sakkas D, Ozenci C-C, Cayli S, Delpiano E, et al. Fertility testing and ICSI sperm selection by hyaluronic acid binding: Clinical and genetic aspects. Reproductive Biomedicine Online. 2007;**14**(5):650-663

[28] Izadi M, Khalili MA, Salehi-Abargouei A, Rezvani ME, Aflatoonian B. Use of zona pellucida-bound spermatozoa as a natural selection in improvement of ICSI outcomes: A systematic review and meta-analysis. Andrologia. 2021;**53**(6):e14022

[29] Izadi M, Khalili MA, Rezvani ME, Anbari F, Maleki B, Woodward B, et al. Sperm selection using zona pellucida–binding enhanced embryo morphokinetic and clinical outcomes in ICSI: A sibling oocytes study. American Journal of Men's Health. 2024;**18**(1):15579883241228236

[30] Nyboe Andersen A, Carlsen E, Loft A. Trends in the use of intracytoplasmatic sperm injection marked variability between countries. Human Reproduction Update. 2008;**14**(6):593-604

[31] Mortimer D. Sperm preparation methods. Journal of Andrology. 2000;**21**(3):357-366

[32] Allamaneni SS, Agarwal A, Rama S, Ranganathan P, Sharma RK. Comparative study on density gradients and swim-up preparation techniques utilizing neat and cryopreserved spermatozoa. Asian Journal of Andrology. 2005;**7**(1):86-92

[33] Rappa K, Samargia J, Sher M, Pino JS, Rodriguez HF, Asghar W. Quantitative analysis of sperm rheotaxis using a microfluidic device. Microfluidics and Nanofluidics. 2018;**22**(9):100

[34] El-Sherry TM, Abdel-Ghani MA, Abdel Hafez HK, Abdelgawad M. Rheotaxis of sperm in fertile and infertile men. Systems Biology in Reproductive Medicine. 2023;**69**(1):57-63

[35] Zhang Z, Liu J, Meriano J, Ru C, Xie S, Luo J, et al. Human sperm rheotaxis: A passive physical process. Scientific Reports. 2016;**6**(1):1-8

[36] Kantsler V, Dunkel J, Blayney M, Goldstein RE. Rheotaxis facilitates upstream navigation of mammalian sperm cells. eLife. 2014;**3**:e02403

[37] Sharma S, Kabir MA, Asghar W. Selection of healthy sperm based on positive rheotaxis using a microfluidic device. The Analyst. 2022;**147**(8):1589-1597

[38] Romero-Aguirregomezcorta J, Laguna-Barraza R, Fernández-González R, Štiavnická M, Ward F, Cloherty J, et al. Sperm selection by rheotaxis improves sperm quality and early embryo development. Reproduction. 2021;**161**(3):343-352

[39] Khodamoradi M, Rafizadeh Tafti S, Mousavi Shaegh SA, Aflatoonian B, Azimzadeh M, Khashayar P. Recent microfluidic innovations for sperm sorting. Chemosensors. 2021;**9**(6):126

[40] Bahat A, Eisenbach M, Tur-Kaspa I. Periovulatory increase in temperature difference within the rabbit oviduct. Human Reproduction. 2005;**20**(8):2118-2121

[41] Bahat A, Eisenbach M. Sperm thermotaxis. Molecular and Cellular Endocrinology. 2006;**252**(1-2):115-119

[42] De Toni L, Dipresa S, Foresta C, Garolla A. Molecular bases of sperm thermotaxis: Old and new knowledges. Protein and Peptide Letters. 2018;**25**(5):446-450

[43] Roy D, Levi K, Kiss V, Nevo R, Eisenbach M. Rhodopsin and melanopsin coexist in mammalian sperm cells and activate different signaling pathways for thermotaxis. Scientific Reports. 2020;**10**(1):112

[44] Pérez-Cerezales S, Boryshpolets S, Afanzar O, Brandis A, Nevo R, Kiss V, et al. Involvement of opsins in mammalian sperm thermotaxis. Scientific Reports. 2015;**5**(1):16146

[45] Yan Y, Zhang B, Fu Q, Wu J, Liu R. A fully integrated biomimetic microfluidic device for evaluation of sperm response to thermotaxis and chemotaxis. Lab on a Chip. 2021;**21**(2):310-318

[46] Guleresi K, Santos Ribeiro S, Reis Soares S, Nunes Gouveia S, Gómez AS. P-076 sperm selection by thermotaxis: A novel technique to enhance assisted reproductive technologies' outcomes. Human Reproduction. 2023;**38**(Supplement_1):dead093. 441

[47] Eisenbach M. Sperm chemotaxis. Reviews of Reproduction. 1999;**4**(1):56-66

[48] Yoshida M, Yoshida K. Sperm chemotaxis and regulation of flagellar movement by $Ca^{2+}$. MHR: Basic Science of Reproductive Medicine. 2011;**17**(8):457-465

[49] Teves ME, Guidobaldi HA, Unates DR, Sanchez R, Miska W, Publicover SJ, et al. Molecular mechanism for human sperm chemotaxis mediated by progesterone. PLoS ONE. 2009;**4**(12):e8211

[50] Friedrich BM, Jülicher F. Chemotaxis of sperm cells. National Academy of Sciences of the United States of America. 2007;**104**(33):13256-13261

[51] Guidobaldi HA, Teves ME, Uñates DR, Anastasía A, Giojalas LC. Progesterone from the cumulus cells is the sperm chemoattractant secreted by the rabbit oocyte cumulus complex. PLoS ONE. 2008;**3**(8):e3040

[52] Eisenbach M. Mammalian sperm chemotaxis and its association with capacitation. Developmental Genetics. 1999;**25**(2):87-94

[53] Xie L, Ma R, Han C, Su K, Zhang Q, Qiu T, et al. Integration of sperm motility and chemotaxis screening with a microchannel-based device. Clinical Chemistry. 2010;**56**(8):1270-1278

[54] Marei W, Ghafari F, Fouladi-Nashta A. Role of hyaluronic acid in maturation and further early embryo development of bovine oocytes. Theriogenology. 2012;**78**(3):670-677

[55] Esterhuizen A, Franken D, Bosman E, Rodrigues F, Van Rensburg J, Van Schouwenburg J, et al. Relationship between human spermatozoa–hyaluronan-binding assay, conventional semen parameters and fertilisation rates in intracytoplasmic spermatozoa injection. Andrologia. 2015;**47**(7):759-764

[56] Parmegiani L, Cognigni GE, Ciampaglia W, Pocognoli P, Marchi F, Filicori M. Efficiency of hyaluronic acid (HA) sperm selection. Journal of Assisted Reproduction and Genetics. 2010;**27**:13-16

[57] Mokanszki A, Tothne EV, Bodnar B, Tandor Z, Molnar Z, Jakab A, et al. Is sperm hyaluronic acid binding ability predictive for clinical success of intracytoplasmic sperm injection: PICSI vs. ICSI? Systems Biology in Reproductive Medicine. 2014;**60**(6):348-354

[58] Huszar G, Ozkavukcu S, Jakab A, Celik-Ozenci C, Sati GL, Cayli S. Hyaluronic acid binding ability of human sperm reflects cellular maturity and fertilizing potential: Selection of sperm for intracytoplasmic sperm injection. Current Opinion in Obstetrics and Gynecology. 2006;**18**(3):260-267

[59] Huang M-T, Lee RK-K, Lu C-H, Chen Y-J, Li S-H, Hwu Y-M. The efficiency of conventional microscopic selection is comparable to the hyaluronic acid binding method in selecting spermatozoa for male infertility patients. Taiwanese Journal of Obstetrics & Gynecology. 2015;**54**(1):48-53

[60] Scaruffi P, Bovis F, Casciano I, Maccarini E, De Leo C, Gazzo I, et al. Hyaluronic acid-sperm selection significantly improves the clinical outcome of couples with previous ICSI cycles failure. Andrology. 2022;**10**(4):677-685

[61] Hozyen M, Hasanen E, Elqusi K, ElTanbouly S, Gamal S, Hussin AG, et al. Reproductive outcomes of different sperm selection techniques for ICSI patients with abnormal sperm DNA fragmentation: A randomized controlled trial. Reproductive Sciences. 2022;**29**(1):220-228

[62] Kim SJ, Kim H, Kim TH, Jeong J, Lee WS, Lyu SW. Effect of sperm selection using hyaluronan on fertilization and quality of cleavage-stage embryos in intracytoplasmic sperm injection (ICSI) cycles of couples with severe teratozoospermia. Gynecological Endocrinology. 2020;**36**(5):456-459

[63] Lefièvre L, Conner S, Salpekar A, Olufowobi O, Ashton P, Pavlovic B, et al. Four zona pellucida glycoproteins are expressed in the human. Human Reproduction. 2004;**19**(7):1580-1586

[64] Gupta SK. The human egg's zona pellucida. Current Topics in Developmental Biology. 2018;**130**:379-411

[65] Menkveld R, Franken DR, Kruger TF, Oehninger S, Hodgen GD. Sperm selection capacity of the human zona pellucida. Molecular Reproduction and Development. 1991;**30**(4):346-352

[66] Leung ET, Lee BK, Lee C-L, Tian X, Lam KK, Li RH, et al. The role of spermatozoa-zona pellucida interaction in selecting fertilization-competent spermatozoa in humans. Frontiers in Endocrinology. 2023;**14**:1135973

[67] Braga DPAF, Iaconelli A Jr, Figueira RCS, Madaschi C, Semião-Francisco L, Borges E Jr. Outcome of ICSI using zona pellucida-bound spermatozoa and conventionally selected spermatozoa. Reproductive Biomedicine Online. 2009;**19**(6):802-807

[68] Ganeva R, Parvanov D, Vasileva M, Nikolova K, Stamenov GS. Higher pregnancy rates after zona pellucida sperm selection. Fertility and Sterility. 2019;**112**(3):e280

[69] Liu F, Qiu Y, Zou Y, Deng Z-H, Yang H. Use of zona pellucida–bound sperm for intracytoplasmic sperm injection produces higher embryo quality and implantation than conventional intracytoplasmic sperm injection. Fertility and Sterility. 2011;**95**(2):815-818

Chapter 4

# A Comparative Analysis of Gradient Centrifugation and Microfluidic Chips for Sperm Selection

*Hale Bayram and Yaprak Donmez Cakil*


## Abstract

A variety of techniques have been employed in the field of sperm selection, including methods based on sperm density, morphological characteristics, motility characteristics, membrane integrity, and surface charge. Among these techniques, the density gradient centrifugation (DGC) method stands out as the most prevalent and widely utilized today. However, this technique involves centrifugation steps that have been linked to oxidative stress and subsequent cellular damage. Consequently, alternatives to DGC are being continuously developed. The recently developed microfluidic chip method has also been implemented for sperm selection in intracytoplasmic sperm injection (ICSI). However, the microfluidic chip method also presents certain disadvantages that must be addressed. This chapter evaluates the advantages and disadvantages of sperm selection methods from the past to the present, with a particular focus on DGC and microfluidic devices.


**Keywords:** density gradient centrifugation, sperm selection, microfluidics, *in vitro* fertilization, intracytoplasmic sperm injection

## 1. Introduction

The global prevalence of infertility in couples of reproductive age is estimated at 15%, with male factor being identified as the primary or contributing cause in 40–50% of cases [1]. Male infertility is often associated with spermatogenic dysfunction, resulting in impaired sperm quality as indicated by aberrant motility, viability, morphology, or concentration, as well as molecular genetic alterations including reduced DNA integrity [1, 2]. The advent of assisted reproductive technology (ART) has enabled individuals with severe male infertility to achieve conception [3, 4]. In particular, intracytoplasmic sperm injection (ICSI) represents a revolutionary method in the field of ART, as fertilization and pregnancy can be achieved even with poor sperm quality and a low sperm count [5].

*In vivo*, high-quality and potentially fertile spermatozoa are separated from seminal plasma by traveling along the cervical mucus in the female genital tract. This process not only selects motile spermatozoa but also induces physiological changes in male germ cells, including capacitation and the acrosome reaction, which enable sperm to gain functional competence [6]. Although ICSI is optimal for treating male factor infertility, it circumvents the biological barriers that ensure the natural selection of gametes. This may result in the fertilization of oocytes with defective spermatozoa, which can lead to developmental failure and reduced ART success rates [5, 7]. Moreover, it also has been observed that the absence of the acrosomal reaction and the persistence of the perinuclear tecta in the sperm head are associated with delayed condensation of DNA during fertilization [8]. Furthermore, ICSI has been linked to an elevated risk of numerous health complications, including premature births, diverse metabolic disorders in the progeny, miscarriages, and congenital malformations [9]. It is therefore crucial to develop efficient procedures and devices to select the most competent sperm, given that ICSI involves injecting a single sperm cell into the oocyte.

A wide range of sperm selection methodologies have been developed, which can be broadly classified based on the selection mechanism, including sperm density, membrane integrity, morphological characteristics, motility characteristics, and surface charge [7, 10]. A number of studies have been conducted with the aim of identifying the optimal methodology for sperm preparation for ART. The objective is to develop a process that is quick, easy to implement, affordable, capable of isolating a large number of motile spermatozoa, and that does not cause damage or physiological changes to the spermatozoa. In addition, the process should eliminate dead sperm, white blood cells, and bacteria, and should also eliminate capacitation-inhibiting

| Method | Method results in | Benefits | Drawbacks |
|---|---|---|---|
| Swim-up | • Morphologically normal and motile sperm. | • Ease of implementation [13].<br>• Extremely cost-effective [6, 7, 11].<br>• No membrane damage and fragmented DNA caused by centrifugation [14]. | • Limited to ejaculates with high volume, high sperm count, and motility [6].<br>• Low yield [15]. |
| Density gradient centrifugation (DGC) | • Morphologically normal and motile sperm. | • High yield [6, 11].<br>• Can be used in combination with swim-up (SU) to improve sperm quality [13].<br>• One of the most widely used techniques in clinical practice [16]. | • Increased mitochondrial damage and decreased probability of pregnancy [14, 17].<br>• Severely damaged spermatozoa due to centrifugation-induced increased ROS and apoptosis during selection with DGC [11, 17]. |
| Migration-sedimentation method | • Morphologically normal sperm with good progressive motility [18]. | • No adverse effects attributed to centrifugation [18].<br>• Extremely cost-effective, practical, and fast [18].<br>• The potential to reduce DNA damage [19]. | • Limited to ejaculates with high volume, high sperm count, and motility; low yield [6, 14, 20].<br>• Requirement for expensive and relatively delicate special tubes [6, 14, 20].<br>• Unsuitable for conventional IVF procedure [11]. |

| Method | Method results in | Benefits | Drawbacks |
|---|---|---|---|
| Hypo-osmotic swelling test (HOST) | • Viable sperm with membrane and DNA integrity [21, 22]. | • Extremely cost-effective<br>• Ease of implementation [11, 23]. | • Spontaneously developed tail swelling in less than 10% of human sperm [11].<br>• Low efficiency with low sperm volume [7]. |
| Magnetic activated cell sorting (MACS) | • Elimination of apoptotic spermatozoa [24, 25]. | • Selection of high-quality sperm with reduced DNA fragmentation [26, 27]. | • Requirement for use in combination with DGC for more efficient selection [11].<br>• Little evidence regarding live birth rates [7, 24, 26]. |
| Fluorescence activated cell sorting (FACS) | • Functional and high-quality sperm with intact DNA [11, 28, 29]. | • Successful chromosomal profiling and identification of segmental aneuploidies [29]. | • High cost and low efficiency [11]. |
| Zeta method | • Mature sperm based on the negative charge of the plasma membrane, known as the Zeta potential, which decreases with capacitation [27].<br>• Selection of morphologically normal sperm with intact DNA [27]. | • Results are obtained with a small amount of semen sample [30].<br>• Fast, cheap and simple [30].<br>• Higher rate of fertilization and higher quality embryos when compared to the DCG method [31]. | • Clinical use not widespread.<br>• Used in addition to other methods because it does not evaluate motility [31]. |
| Laser-assisted immotile sperm selection (LAISS) | • Motile sperm | • Fast, no centrifugation required [32].<br>• Only technique available to detect viable sperm in patients with primary cilia dyskinesia (PCD) [32, 33]. | • High cost [11].<br>• Cause membrane rupture and increase ROS levels [34].<br>• Experience required [11]. |
| Microfluidics | • Morphologically normal and motile sperm. | • Ease of use.<br>• Controlled and automated process [11].<br>• Eliminates damage caused by centrifugation and provides a higher euploid embryo formation rate [35–37].<br>• A selection environment that mimics *in vivo* and behaves similarly to cervical mucus with little or no adverse effects [38]. | • The complexity of the devices in use [11].<br>• Low efficiency with low sperm count [7]. |

**Table 1.**
*Benefits and drawbacks of sperm selection methods.*

factors and toxic substances such as reactive oxygen species (ROS) [11, 12]. However, a review of the available literature reveals a considerable degree of inconsistency in the outcomes reported. The most commonly used methods for sperm selection, along with their advantages and disadvantages, are listed in **Table 1**.

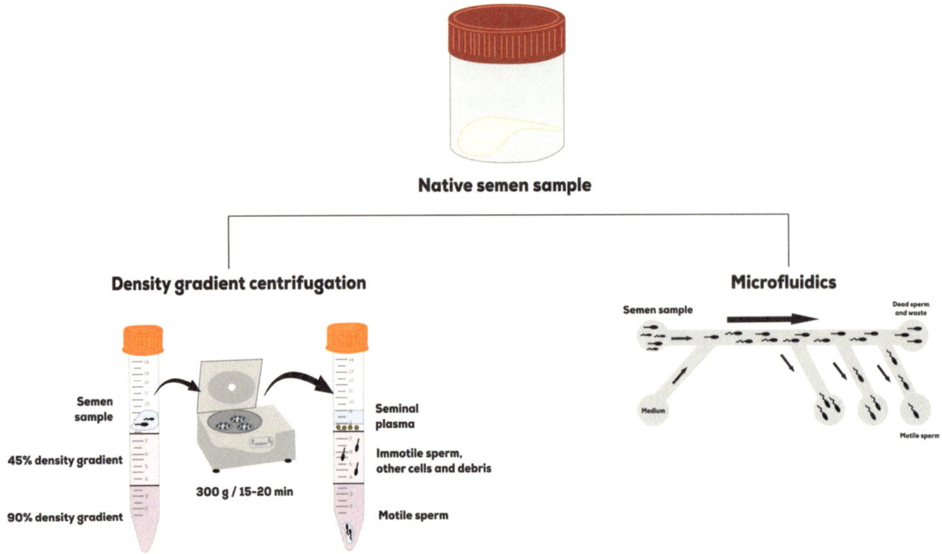


**Figure 1.**
*Schematics of sperm preparation by density gradient separation and microfluidic technology (created using Adobe Illustrator version 28.3, USA).*

Of these techniques, gradient centrifugation, which selects sperm according to their density and motility, is widely used in clinical practice. It should be noted, however, that this technique involves centrifugation steps that are known to cause oxidative stress and thus damage cells. Therefore, alternatives to gradient centrifugation are constantly being developed. The recently developed microfluidics technology has been introduced as a powerful platform for sperm selection in ICSI procedures. However, microfluidic devices also present some challenges that need to be addressed. This chapter will provide an objective analysis of the benefits and drawbacks of sperm selection methods, with a particular focus on DGC and microfluidic devices, comparing past and present approaches (**Figure 1**).

## 2. Density gradient centrifugation for sperm separation

Centrifugation is a process that is employed in a variety of fields and is based on the spinning of a mixture at a certain speed to separate its components. There are three principal types of centrifugation, namely differential centrifugation, DGC, and ultracentrifugation [39]. DGC is a method used since the 1950s in numerous fields, including biology and medicine, for the separation of cells, subcellular organelles, and macromolecules based on their size, shape, viscosity, or density of the medium through rotation at a specific speed [40–42].

Among the various standardized protocols for sperm selection for IVF treatments in andrology laboratories, DGC is a method that has been recommended by the World Health Organization (WHO) [43]. DGC allows for the separation of spermatozoa based on their density and motility by placing seminal plasma on a continuous or discontinuous density gradient. In a continuous gradient, the density increases gradually from the top to the bottom of the gradient. In contrast, a discontinuous gradient exhibits distinct boundaries between each layer [7, 11, 44]. Commonly, a semen sample is placed on top of two superimposed solutions of varying densities for the purpose of sperm separation and then subjected to centrifugation for approximately 15–20 minutes. All sperm cells pass through the gradients, but the highly motile spermatozoa migrate to the bottom of the tube, moving vigorously rather than being subjected to centrifugal kinetics. This results in the formation of a pellet at the bottom of the tube. In contrast, dead cells, immotile cells, and debris remain between the gradients [45]. In addition, the densities of immobile (1.06 g/mL) and immature (1.09 g/mL) spermatozoa are lower than that of a motile, mature spermatozoon (1.10 g/mL) [46]. Consequently, following centrifugation, morphologically abnormal spermatozoa are concentrated between the upper and lower layers, and leukocytes and cell debris are between the seminal plasma and the upper layer. Motile and mature spermatozoa form a pellet at the bottom of the tube [47].

A variety of gradient media have been formulated with the objective of providing an ideal medium for separation. A commercial DGC medium, Percoll® gradient, consisting of polyvinylpyrrolidone (PVP)-coated silica particles, was widely used until it was discontinued by its manufacturer in 1996 due to concerns about the toxicity caused by endotoxin contamination [6]. Further studies focusing on the safety of PVP for its clinical use demonstrated the detrimental effects on sperm function, fertilization success, and early embryonic development in patients undergoing ICSI [48]. PureSperm® and Isolate® have emerged as replacements for Percoll® and have demonstrated effective separation capabilities due to the intrinsic properties of colloidal silica, including the absence of an osmotic effect, the ability to provide high specific gravity and low viscosity. In contrast to Percoll®, these two commercial products utilize silane-coated colloidal silica [49].

Today, a diverse array of DGC media are now extensively utilized in the context of infertility treatment. A multitude of studies have been conducted to comparatively assess the efficacy of various media to obtain spermatozoa that exhibit optimal motility and morphologic normality, while overcoming toxicity, osmotic pressure changes, and penetration into particles. The classical density gradient medium sucrose was unsuccessful due to its high osmolality and viscosity [50]. Ficoll, a synthetic polymer of sucrose, was introduced to address the issue of high osmotic pressures. Recently, the combination of the Ficoll-400 density gradient method with the swim-up technique has been proposed as an effective approach for sperm preparation prior to ART [51]. Iodinated compounds, including Nycodenz® and the dimeric form Iodixanol®, have also been demonstrated to be effective for the selection of motile spermatozoa [52, 53]. IxaPrep®, a polysucrose medium containing Iodixanol, demonstrated superior efficacy in recovering motile spermatozoa from both normal and subnormal semen samples compared to Percoll. Furthermore, it was reported that the production of nitric oxide was lower in semen samples that had been separated using IxaPrep compared to those that had been prepared using Percoll [54]. Another study was conducted to evaluate the sperm quality following sperm separation using three commonly employed commercial media: PureCeption®, ISolate®, and SpermGrad-125®. While the sperm treated with Isolate and SpermGrad-125 demonstrated superior motility, the DNA damage rates were found to be comparable across all three gradients [55]. A recent study compared the sperm recovery rate following sperm separation with ISolate and GV Gradiente, another method based on silane-coated colloidal silica. No differences were identified between the methods in retrieving motile sperm [45].

The DGC method offers a series of advantages that have contributed to its widespread use in the clinical setting. A number of studies have demonstrated that DGC effectively eliminates leukocytes and immature spermatozoa with abnormal morphology, which are the primary sources of endogenous ROS in semen. Moreover, it has been shown that this method yields spermatozoa that are normal in terms of motility [43, 47]. Spermatozoa obtained by DGC demonstrated increased levels of hyperactivation and tyrosine phosphorylation, indicating a higher degree of capacitation [43]. In addition, DGC is a time-saving technique, as it requires only about 15–20 minutes of centrifugation compared to 1 hour of incubation for the swim-up method. The method is straightforward to perform under sterile conditions, which makes it a highly feasible approach [56].

It should be noted that the DGC method also has limitations. The rate of DNA fragmentation has been shown to increase during sperm separation by the DGC method due to centrifugation. Research indicates that centrifuge-based separation techniques may potentially damage sperm, which could result in iatrogenic failed pregnancies [14]. Some studies reported that a sequential combination of DGC and the swim-up method has the potential to mitigate DNA damage [57, 58]. Nevertheless, these classical methods are considered inadequate because they rely solely on separation mechanisms based on morphology and mobility. The DGC method has recently been compared with microfluidic methods, which have been proposed as an alternative to centrifuge-based techniques. Microfluidics has been demonstrated to reduce DNA damage and the production of ROS [59], while also leading to enhanced sperm motility and blastocyst quality in comparison to DGC [44]. The following section presents a discussion on the use of microfluidic systems for sperm sorting in the context of ART, with an evaluation of the clinical outcomes.

## 3. Microfluidics for sperm separation

The use of microfluidic technology for sperm separation represents a novel and efficacious approach that has been developed as an alternative to traditional techniques. In 2017, Smith and Takayama published one of the first successful studies demonstrating the use and efficacy of microfluidics for human sperm selection [35]. This technique has since become a powerful system for sperm selection, whereby the physiological conditions of the female reproductive system, such as pH and temperature, are simulated [60].

The term "microfluidics" is used to describe the study of fluid behavior at the sub-microliter level ($10^{-9}$–$10^{-18}$ liters) and its measurement with a variety of microfluidic devices. It is a technological system that processes or manipulates small quantities of liquids using micrometer-sized channels. As a multidisciplinary and interdisciplinary field, microfluidics encompasses engineering, physics, chemistry, biology, and biotechnology [60]. In the early stages of microfluidic device development, glass and silicon were the primary materials employed. However, their high cost presented a significant obstacle. Subsequently, polymers such as polydimethylsiloxane (PDMS) and thermoplastics were used instead of glass and silicon in microfluidic technology [61].

Initially introduced in the early 1990s, microfluidic technologies offer several advantages, including the ability to analyze very small sample sizes, high resolution and sensitivity, high detection capability, low cost, and a short analysis time [35, 62]. This technology is employed in a number of fields, including, control of fluid transport, cell analysis, and drug delivery systems as well as in the field of ART for the collection and isolation of sperm [61]. Furthermore, microfluidics devices are utilized in a multitude of additional stages of ART, including embryo culture, cryopreservation, oocyte separation, gamete fertilization, and embryo quality analysis [60].

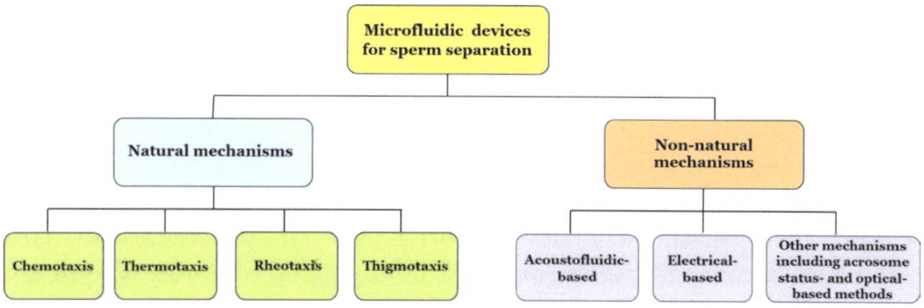


**Figure 2.**
*The principal mechanisms utilized in microfluidic devices for sperm separation (created in draw.io (ENG)).*

The use of microfluidics has been demonstrated to eliminate the mechanical stress associated with centrifugation on sperm in several studies [59]. Moreover, the microfluidic technique has been reported to facilitate high forward motility and the production of high-quality embryos [44]. Additionally, it has been shown to enhance the proportion of normal sperm morphology and significantly reduce the percentage of DNA damage compared to centrifugation [59, 63–67].

Various microfluidic devices have been designed to separate sperm with different mechanisms, which can be grouped into two main categories, natural and non-natural methods [68], as shown in **Figure 2**.

### 3.1 Natural mechanisms

The female reproductive system has several mechanisms to guide sperm to the site of fertilization [68]. Various microfluidic devices have been constructed with the objective of separating spermatozoa according to the aforementioned natural mechanisms, including movement directed by a chemical gradient (chemotaxis), movement directed by a thermal gradient (thermotaxis), swimming against the flow (rheotaxis), and boundary-following behavior (thigmotaxis) [68–70].

Chemotaxis is one of the natural mechanisms that enables sperm to navigate a chemical gradient secreted by the female genital system. It is known to be the primary guiding mechanism during the final phase of the journey through the female reproductive tract, allowing approximately 10% of motile spermatozoa to reach the oocyte [68, 71, 72]. Microfluidics is frequently utilized to emulate this natural guidance mechanism for the screening and separation of human spermatozoa [68, 71, 73]. Progesterone, allurin, natriuretic peptide type C (NPPC), heparin, antithrombin III, acetylcholine (ACh), adrenaline, and calcitonin are defined as natural sperm chemoattractants. Among these, progesterone and ACh have been employed to establish a gradient concentration for the separation of spermatozoa [74, 75]. It is hypothesized that the progesterone produced by the cells of the cumulus creates a gradient from the center to the periphery of the cell mass [72, 76]. ACh has been demonstrated to originate from follicular fluid in the oviducts during ovulation and is postulated to be involved in the induction of chemotaxis due to the presence of ACh receptors on sperm [77].

Another significant mechanism is thermotaxis, which is a longer-range selection mechanism compared to chemotaxis and guides sperm along a temperature gradient within the oviduct [71, 78, 79]. Spermatozoa exhibit thermotactic behavior, moving toward increasing temperature. Recently, it has been demonstrated that thermotactic motility is reduced in spermatozoa with impaired DNA integrity, while motile spermatozoa with high DNA integrity exhibit more pronounced thermotactic behavior, thus reinforcing sperm selection by eliminating sperm with DNA fragmentation [80].

The term "rheotaxis" is derived from the Greek word for flow regulation and refers to the phenomenon of spermatozoa aligning their swimming direction with or against fluid flow. The controversy surrounding sperm rheotaxis persists regarding whether it is a passive or active process. However, recent experimental studies have indicated that it is, in fact, a passive process [81]. This process allows mature and motile spermatozoa to travel through the oviduct, and reach the oocyte, thereby facilitating fertilization [82]. During coitus, fluids are secreted by the female genital tract, including the oviducts. These fluids are thought to create a fluid flow along the reproductive tract providing clues for spermatozoa traveling in the opposite direction to the fluid flow toward the uterus [81].

Rheotaxis-based microfluidic devices have been developed to simulate fluid flows and micro-grooves in the female genital tract. The swimming behavior of sperm cells when encountering corrugated and smooth channels has been observed and isolated sperm have shown high motility. A number of studies have been conducted with these microfluidic devices, yielding results that indicate a reduction in DNA damage [83].

Spermatozoa are cells that are capable of active swimming due to the presence of a flagellum. The boundary-following behavior of motile spermatozoa is a defining characteristic of this ability. Spermatozoa develop boundary-following behavior to reach the oocyte through a challenging course in the female genital tract, which is full of labyrinths, narrow passages, complex pathways, and viscous fluids [71]. The studies indicated that the motility of spermatozoa increased and the rate of DNA damage decreased in microfluidic chips containing a thigmotaxis mechanism in conjunction with rheotaxis, in comparison to the rheotaxis method alone [84].

### 3.2 Non-natural mechanisms

A variety of non-natural mechanisms for sperm separation have been developed, including acoustofluidic-based methods and electrical-based methods such as electrophoresis and dielectrophoresis. Acoustic flow refers to the fluid motion produced by the interaction of sound waves with a fluid medium. Acoustic microfluidics, which employs an ultrasonic bubble oscillation mechanism, is the preferred method due to its minimal physiological impact on biological samples, its versatility in a range of applications, and its straightforward implementation [65]. The selection of the wave frequencies used in acoustic-based microfluidics is crucial, as depending on the wave frequencies, sperm separation reveals contradictory results [65, 85].

Electrical-based electrophoresis and dielectrophoresis are frequently used methods in biotechnology and medicine for the manipulation of microscale bioparticles, including cell separation, sorting, and capture [86]. Electrophoresis can induce the movement of charged particles in cells through a uniform electric field in a fluid, while dielectrophoresis employs a non-uniform alternating current electric field to exert force on dielectric particles [71]. The advancement of electrode-based microfluidic devices allows for the acquisition of real-time data for both spermatozoa selection and single-cell analysis. In comparison to chemotaxis, thermotaxis, and even motility-based sperm selection, electrical-based sperm selection offers the greatest control and can be modified by immediate system intervention [87].

In addition to the aforementioned methods, studies have demonstrated the effectiveness of different microfluidics platforms utilizing diverse selection mechanisms. However, there is a need for further research on these platforms in the context of ART [68].

While recent studies have demonstrated the superiority of microfluidic technologies over conventional methods in reducing centrifugation-induced mechanical stress and subsequent DNA damage, it remains crucial to evaluate the reproductive outcomes to ascertain the efficacy of microfluidic devices in clinical settings. A recent study demonstrated that microfluidic sperm selection markedly enhanced the proportion of spermatozoa with an intact genome, contributing to higher embryo euploidy and implantation rates and resulting in increased term pregnancies in comparison to DGC [88]. Similarly, sperm preparation with microfluidics demonstrated superior results compared to DGC, with higher blastocyst formation, utilization, and euploidy rates in patients undergoing ICSI [89]. A number of other studies also reported enhanced laboratory parameters and clinical outcomes with the application of microfluidics technology prior to ART [59]. Some studies have indicated that the use of microfluidics may result in a notable increase in pregnancy rates only in older patients [90, 91].

Conversely, a recent systematic review and meta-analysis compiling 13 studies and comparing the efficacy of microfluidics with conventional sperm preparation techniques, including DGC, indicated a marginal improvement in ART outcomes, though this was not statistically significant [92].

## 4. Conclusion

In clinical settings, the rapidity, cost-effectiveness, ease of learning, and high reproducibility of the sperm selection technique are of significant concern. However, each sperm separation method has its own set of advantages and disadvantages, and there is not yet sufficient data to demonstrate that any of them can be considered the gold standard. Microfluidic technologies offer significant advantages to DGC, including reduced DNA damage and the prevention of centrifugation-induced mechanical stress [38, 93]. The controlled and automated process simplifies sperm selection and reduces the risk of errors. The currently available evidence suggests that microfluidics may be a promising option for optimizing success in ICSI treatments. Nevertheless, further studies are required to reduce its cost and clarify its potential for ARTs.

## Conflict of interest

The authors declare no conflict of interest.

## Author details

Hale Bayram and Yaprak Donmez Cakil*
Department of Histology and Embryology, Faculty of Medicine, Maltepe University, Istanbul, Türkiye

*Address all correspondence to: yaprak.cakil@maltepe.edu.tr

## References

[1] Amano K, Oigawa S, Ichizawa K, Tokuda Y, Unagami M, Sekiguchi M, et al. Swim-up method is superior to density gradient centrifugation for preserving sperm DNA integrity during sperm processing. Reproductive Medicine and Biology. 2024;**23**(1):e12562

[2] Berteli TS, Da Broi MG, Martins WP, Ferriani RA, Navarro PA. Magnetic-activated cell sorting before density gradient centrifugation improves recovery of high-quality spermatozoa. Andrology. 2017;**5**(4):776-782

[3] Mazzilli R, Rucci C, Vaiarelli A, Cimadomo D, Ubaldi FM, Foresta C, et al. Male factor infertility and assisted reproductive technologies: Indications, minimum access criteria and outcomes. Journal of Endocrinological Investigation. 2023;**46**(6):1079-1085

[4] Tournaye H. Male factor infertility and ART. Asian Journal of Andrology. 2012;**14**(1):103-108

[5] Oseguera-López I, Ruiz-Díaz S, Ramos-Ibeas P, Pérez-Cerezales S. Novel techniques of Sperm selection for improving IVF and ICSI outcomes. Frontiers in Cell and Development Biology. 2019;**7**:298

[6] Henkel RR, Schill WB. Sperm preparation for ART. Reproductive Biology and Endocrinology. 2003;**1**(1):108

[7] Baldini D, Ferri D, Baldini GM, Lot D, Catino A, Vizziello D, et al. Sperm selection for ICSI: Do we have a winner? Cells. 2021;**10**(12):3566

[8] D'Onofrio BM, Rickert ME, Frans E, Kuja-Halkola R, Almqvist C, Sjölander A, et al. Paternal age at childbearing and offspring psychiatric and academic morbidity. JAMA Psychiatry. 2014;**71**(4):432

[9] Sánchez-Calabuig MJ, López-Cardona AP, Fernández-González R, Ramos-Ibeas P, Fonseca Balvís N, Laguna-Barraza R, et al. Potential health risks associated to ICSI: Insights from animal models and strategies for a safe procedure. Frontiers in Public Health. 2014;**2**:241. Available from: http://journal.frontiersin.org/article/10.3389/fpubh.2014.00241/abstract

[10] Vaughan DA, Sakkas D. Sperm selection methods in the 21st century. Biology of Reproduction. 2019;**101**(6):1076-1082

[11] Marzano G, Chiriacò MS, Primiceri E, Dell'Aquila ME, Ramalho-Santos J, Zara V, et al. Sperm selection in assisted reproduction: A review of established methods and cutting-edge possibilities. Biotechnology Advances. 2020;**40**:107498

[12] Pedrosa ML, Furtado MH, Ferreira MCF, Carneiro MM. Sperm selection in IVF: The long and winding road from bench to bedside. JBRA Assisted Reproduction. 2020;**24**(3):332-339

[13] Hsu CT, Lee CI, Lin FS, Wang FZ, Chang HC, Wang TE, et al. Live motile sperm sorting device for enhanced sperm-fertilization competency: Comparative analysis with density-gradient centrifugation and microfluidic sperm sorting. Journal of Assisted Reproduction and Genetics. 2023;**40**(8):1855-1864

[14] Meitei HY, Uppangala S, Sharan K, Chandraguthi SG, Radhakrishnan A, Kalthur G, et al. A simple, centrifugation-

free, sperm-sorting device eliminates the risks of centrifugation in the swim-up method while maintaining functional competence and DNA integrity of selected spermatozoa. Reproductive Sciences. 2021;**28**(1):134-143

[15] Björndahl L, Apolikhin O, Baldi E, Barratt CLR, Festin MPR, Kirkman-Brown JC, et al., editors. WHO Laboratory Manual for the Examination and Processing of Human Semen. 6th ed. Geneva: World Health Organization; 2021. Available from: https://apps.who.int/iris/handle/10665/343208

[16] De Martin H, Miranda EP, Cocuzza MS, Monteleone PAA. Density gradient centrifugation and swim-up for ICSI: Useful, unsafe, or just unsuitable? Journal of Assisted Reproduction and Genetics. 2019;**36**(12):2421-2423

[17] Muratori M, Tarozzi N, Carpentiero F, Danti S, Perrone FM, Cambi M, et al. Sperm selection with density gradient centrifugation and swim up: Effect on DNA fragmentation in viable spermatozoa. Scientific Reports. 2019;**9**(1):7492

[18] Kiratli S, Yuncu M, Kose K, Ozkavukcu S. A comparative evaluation of migration sedimentation method for sperm preparation. Systems Biology in Reproductive Medicine. 2018;**64**(2):122-129

[19] Ramos VB, Cipriani DDC, Araújo ES, Salvador RA, Senn AP, Frajblat M, et al. Sperm selection using three semen processing techniques. JBRA Assisted Reproduction. 2015;**19**(4):223-226

[20] Tea NT, Jondet M, Scholler R. A 'migration-gravity sedimentation' method for collecting motile spermatozoa from human semen. In: Harrison RF, Bonnar J, Thompson W, editors. In Vitro Fertilization, Embryo Transfer and Early Pregnancy. Dordrecht: Springer Netherlands; 1984. pp. 117-120. Available from: http://link.springer.com/10.1007/978-94-011-8132-7_21

[21] Bloch A, Rogers EJ, Nicolas C, Martin-Denavit T, Monteiro M, Thomas D, et al. Detailed cell-level analysis of sperm nuclear quality among the different hypo-osmotic swelling test (HOST) classes. Journal of Assisted Reproduction and Genetics. 2021;**38**(9):2491-2499

[22] Charehjooy N, Najafi MH, Tavalaee M, Deemeh MR, Azadi L, Shiravi AH, et al. Selection of sperm based on hypo-osmotic swelling may improve ICSI outcome: A preliminary prospective clinical trial. International Journal of Fertility and Sterility. 2014;**8**(1):21-28

[23] Jeyendran RS, Van Der Ven HH, Perez-Pelaez M, Crabo BG, Zaneveld LJD. Development of an assay to assess the functional integrity of the human sperm membrane and its relationship to other semen characteristics. Reproduction. 1984;**70**(1):219-228

[24] Cakar Z, Cetinkaya B, Aras D, Koca B, Ozkavukcu S, Kaplanoglu İ, et al. Does combining magnetic-activated cell sorting with density gradient or swim-up improve sperm selection? Journal of Assisted Reproduction and Genetics. 2016;**33**(8):1059-1065

[25] Czétány P, Balló A, Márk L, Török A, Szántó Á, Máté G. An alternative application of magnetic-activated cell sorting: CD45 and CD235a based purification of semen and testicular tissue samples. International Journal of Molecular Sciences. 2024;**25**(7):3627

[26] Nadalini M, Tarozzi N, Di Santo M, Borini A. Annexin V magnetic-activated

cell sorting versus swim-up for the selection of human sperm in ART: Is the new approach better then the traditional one? Journal of Assisted Reproduction and Genetics. 2014;**31**(8):1045-1051

[27] Zahedi A, Tavalaee M, Deemeh MR, Azadi L, Fazilati M, Nasr-Esfahani MH. Zeta potential vs apoptotic marker: Which is more suitable for ICSI sperm selection? Journal of Assisted Reproduction and Genetics. 2013;**30**(9):1181-1186

[28] Funaro MG, Kim HH, Mazel S, Bolyakov A, Goldstein M, Schlegel PN, et al. A novel sorting technology allows for highly efficient selection of sperm without chromatin damage. Systems Biology in Reproductive Medicine. 2013;**59**(3):172-177

[29] Tran QT, Jatsenko T, Poolamets O, Tšuiko O, Lubenets D, Reimand T, et al. Chromosomal scan of single sperm cells by combining fluorescence-activated cell sorting and next-generation sequencing. Journal of Assisted Reproduction and Genetics. 2019;**36**(1):91-97

[30] Ionov M, Gontarek W, Bryszewska M. Zeta potential technique for analyzing semen quality. MethodsX. 2020;7:100895

[31] Nasr, Esfahani MH, Deemeh MR, Tavalaee M, Sekhavati MH, Gourabi H. Zeta sperm selection improves pregnancy rate and alters sex ratio in male factor infertility patients: A double-blind, randomized clinical trial. International Journal of Fertility and Sterility. 2016;**10**(2):253-260. DOI: 10.22074/ijfs.2016.4917

[32] Aktan TM, Montag M, Duman S, Gorkemli H, Rink K, Yurdakul T. Use of a laser to detect viable but immotile spermatozoa. Andrologia. 2004;**36**(6):366-369

[33] Gerber PA, Kruse R, Hirchenhain J, Krüssel JS, Neumann NJ. Pregnancy after laser-assisted selection of viable spermatozoa before intracytoplasmatic sperm injection in a couple with male primary cilia dyskinesia. Fertility and Sterility. 2008;**89**(6):1826.e9-1826.e12

[34] Montag M. Laser-induced immobilization and plasma membrane permeabilization in human spermatozoa. Human Reproduction. 2000;**15**(4):846-852

[35] Smith GD, Takayama S. Application of microfluidic technologies to human assisted reproduction. Molecular Human Reproduction. 2017;**23**(4):257-268

[36] Parrella A, Choi D, Keating D, Rosenwaks Z, Palermo GD. A microfluidic device for selecting the most progressively motile spermatozoa yields a higher rate of euploid embryos. Fertility and Sterility. 2018;**110**(4):e342

[37] Zhang B, Yin TL, Yang J. A novel microfluidic device for selecting human sperm to increase the proportion of morphologically normal, motile sperm with uncompromised DNA integrity. Analytical Methods. 2015;7(14):5981-5988

[38] Olatunji O, More A. A review of the impact of microfluidics technology on sperm selection technique. Cureus. 2022. Available from: https://www.cureus.com/articles/104256-a-review-of-the-impact-of-microfluidics-technology-on-sperm-selection-technique

[39] Olatunde A, Obidola MS, Tijjani H. Chapter 3—Centrifugation techniques. In: Egbuna C, Patrick-Iwuanyanwu KC, Shah MA, Ifemeje JC, Rasul A, editors. Analytical Techniques in Biosciences. United Kingdom: Academic Press; 2022. pp. 43-58. Available from: https://www.sciencedirect.com/science/article/pii/B9780128226544000087

[40] Brakke MK. Density gradient centrifugation: A new separation

technique 1. Journal of the American Chemical Society. 1951;**73**(4):1847-1848

[41] Harwood R. Cell separation by gradient centrifugation. International Review of Cytology. 1974;**38**:369-403

[42] Majekodunmi SO. A review on centrifugation in the pharmaceutical industry. American Journal of Biomedical Engineering. 2015;**5**(2):67-78

[43] Hernández-Silva G, López-Torres AS, Maldonado-Rosas I, Mata-Martínez E, Larrea F, Torres-Flores V, et al. Effects of semen processing on sperm function: Differences between swim-up and density gradient centrifugation. World Journal of Men's Health. 2021;**39**(4):740

[44] Guler C, Melil S, Ozekici U, Donmez Cakil Y, Selam B, Cincik M. Sperm selection and embryo development: A comparison of the density gradient centrifugation and microfluidic chip sperm preparation methods in patients with astheno-teratozoospermia. Life. 2021;**11**(9):933

[45] Fernandes NDS, Silva CGD, Panizzon GP, Cerialle PMA, Câmara VCM, Radaelli MR, et al. Comparative sperm recovery rate after density gradient centrifugation with two media for in vitro fertilization. JBRA Assisted Reproduction. 2023;**27**(1):25-28

[46] Oshio S, Kaneko S, Iizuka R, Mohri H. Effects of gradient centrifugation on human sperm. Archives of Andrology. 1987;**19**(1):85-93

[47] Takeshima T, Yumura Y, Kuroda S, Kawahara T, Uemura H, Iwasaki A. Effect of density gradient centrifugation on reactive oxygen species in human semen. Systems Biology in Reproductive Medicine. 2017;**63**(3):192-198

[48] Kato Y, Nagao Y. Effect of polyvinylpyrrolidone on sperm function and early embryonic development following intracytoplasmic sperm injection in human assisted reproduction. Reproductive Medicine and Biology. 2012;**11**(4):165-176

[49] Mortimer D. Sperm preparation methods. Journal of Andrology. 2000;**21**(3):357-366

[50] Pertoft H. Fractionation of cells and subcellular particles with Percoll. Journal of Biochemical and Biophysical Methods. 2000;**44**(1-2):1-30

[51] Highland H, Rishika AS, Almira SS, Kanthi PB. Ficoll-400 density gradient method as an effective sperm preparation technique for assisted reproductive techniques. Journal of Human Reproductive Sciences. 2016;**9**(3):194

[52] Gellert-Mortimer ST, Clarke GN, Baker HWG, Hyne RV, Johnston WIH. Evaluation of Nycodenz and Percoll density gradients for the selection of motile human spermatozoa. Fertility and Sterility. 1988;**49**(2):335-341

[53] Harrison K. Iodixanol as a density gradient medium for the isolation of motile spermatozoa. Journal of Assisted Reproduction and Genetics. 1997;**14**(7):385-387

[54] Makkar G, Ng HY, Yeung SB, Ho PC. Comparison of two colloidal silica-based sperm separation media with a non–silica-based medium. Fertility and Sterility. 1999;**72**(5):796-802

[55] Malvezzi H, Sharma R, Agarwal A, Abuzenadah AM, Abu-Elmagd M. Sperm quality after density gradient centrifugation with three commercially available media: A controlled

trial. Reproductive Biology and Endocrinology. 2014;**12**(1):121

[56] Ali AH, Ajina T, Ali MB, Mehdi M. Efficacy of density gradient centrifugation technique (DGC) in enhancing sperm cell DNA quality for assisted reproductive technique. Middle East Fertility Society Journal. 2022;**27**(1):22

[57] Ghumman S, Adiga SK, Upadhya D, Kalthur G, Jayaraman V, Rao SB, et al. Combination of swim-up and density gradient separation methods effectively eliminate DNA damaged sperm. Journal of the Turkish-German Gynecological Association. 2011;**12**(3):148-152

[58] Jamil M, Debbarh H, Kabit A, Ennaji M, Koumba L, Kaarouch I, et al. Comparison between density gradient centrifugation method, an extended version of the horizontal swim up method and the combination of both for sperm selection. Obstetrics & Gynecology Science. 2023;**66**(3):221-229

[59] Anbari F, Khalili MA, Sultan Ahamed AM, Mangoli E, Nabi A, Dehghanpour F, et al. Microfluidic sperm selection yields higher sperm quality compared to conventional method in ICSI program: A pilot study. Systems Biology in Reproductive Medicine. 2021;**67**(2):137-143

[60] Alias AB, Huang HY, Yao DJ. A review on microfluidics: An aid to assisted reproductive technology. Molecules. 2021;**26**(14):4354

[61] Thapa S, Heo YS. Microfluidic technology for in vitro fertilization (IVF). JMST Advances. 2019;**1**(1-2):1-11

[62] Whitesides GM. The origins and the future of microfluidics. Nature. 2006;**442**(7101):368-373

[63] Huang HY, Huang PW, Yao DJ. Enhanced efficiency of sorting sperm motility utilizing a microfluidic chip. Microsystem Technologies. 2017;**23**(2):305-312

[64] Pujol A, García-Peiró A, Ribas-Maynou J, Lafuente R, Mataró D, Vassena R. A microfluidic sperm-sorting device reduces the proportion of sperm with double-stranded DNA fragmentation. Zygote. 2022;**30**(2):200-205

[65] Saeidpour Z, Bouloorchi M, Javadizadeh S, Habibi Z, Badieirostami M. Acoustofluidic-based motile sperm isolation using microvortices. In: 2023 30th National and 8th International Iranian Conference on Biomedical Engineering (ICBME). Tehran, Islamic Republic of Iran: IEEE; 2023. pp. 115-120. Available from: https://ieeexplore.ieee.org/document/10488517/

[66] Schulte RT, Chung YK, Ohl DA, Takayama S, Smith GD. Microfluidic sperm sorting device provides a novel method for selecting motile sperm with higher DNA integrity. Fertility and Sterility. 2007;**88**:S76

[67] Shirota K, Yotsumoto F, Itoh H, Obama H, Hidaka N, Nakajima K, et al. Separation efficiency of a microfluidic sperm sorter to minimize sperm DNA damage. Fertility and Sterility. 2016;**105**(2):315-321.e1

[68] Bouloorchi Tabalvandani M, Saeidpour Z, Habibi Z, Javadizadeh S, Firoozabadi SA, Badieirostami M. Microfluidics as an emerging paradigm for assisted reproductive technology: A sperm separation perspective. Biomedical Microdevices. 2024;**26**(2):23

[69] Berendsen JTW. Microfluidic Spermatozoa Selection for Clinical

Applications. Enschede: University of Twente; 2019

[70] Samuel R, Feng H, Jafek A, Despain D, Jenkins T, Gale B. Microfluidic—Based sperm sorting & analysis for treatment of male infertility. Translational Andrology and Urology. 2018;**7**(S3):S336-S347

[71] Jahangiri AR, Ziarati N, Dadkhah E, Bucak MN, Rahimizadeh P, Shahverdi A, et al. Microfluidics: The future of sperm selection in assisted reproduction. Andrology. 2024;**12**:1236-1252

[72] Kaupp UB, Kashikar ND, Weyand I. Mechanisms of sperm chemotaxis. Annual Review of Physiology. 2008;**70**(1):93-117

[73] Huang J, Chen H, Li N, Zhao Y. Emerging microfluidic technologies for sperm sorting. Engineered Regeneration. 2023;**4**(2):161-169

[74] Berendsen JTW, Kruit SA, Atak N, Willink E, Segerink LI. Flow-free microfluidic device for quantifying chemotaxis in spermatozoa. Analytical Chemistry. 2020;**92**(4):3302-3306

[75] Ko YJ, Maeng JH, Hwang SY, Ahn Y. Design, fabrication, and testing of a microfluidic device for thermotaxis and chemotaxis assays of sperm. SLAS Technology. 2018;**23**(6):507-515

[76] Teves ME, Guidobaldi HA, Uñates DR, Sanchez R, Miska W, Publicover SJ, et al. Molecular mechanism for human sperm chemotaxis mediated by progesterone. PLoS ONE. 2009;**4**(12):e8211

[77] Bhagwat S, Sontakke S, Deekshith K, Parte P, Jadhav S. Chemotactic behavior of spermatozoa captured using a microfluidic chip. Biomicrofluidics. 2018;**12**(2):024112

[78] Bahat A, Caplan SR, Eisenbach M. Thermotaxis of human sperm cells in extraordinarily shallow temperature gradients over a wide range. PLoS ONE. 2012;**7**(7):e41915

[79] Pérez-Cerezales S, Bermejo-Álvarez P. TRPV1: A channel for mammalian sperm thermotaxis? Translational Cancer Research. 2017;**6**(S2):S395-S398

[80] Pérez-Cerezales S, Laguna-Barraza R, De Castro AC, Sánchez-Calabuig MJ, Cano-Oliva E, De Castro-Pita FJ, et al. Sperm selection by thermotaxis improves ICSI outcome in mice. Scientific Reports. 2018;**8**(1):2902

[81] Zhang Z, Liu J, Meriano J, Ru C, Xie S, Luo J, et al. Human sperm rheotaxis: A passive physical process. Scientific Reports. 2016;**6**(1):23553

[82] Sarbandi IR, Lesani A, Moghimi Zand M, Nosrati R. Rheotaxis-based sperm separation using a biomimicry microfluidic device. Scientific Reports. 2021;**11**(1):18327

[83] Heydari A, Zabetian Targhi M, Halvaei I, Nosrati R. A novel microfluidic device with parallel channels for sperm separation using spermatozoa intrinsic behaviors. Scientific Reports. 2023;**13**(1):1185

[84] Zeaei S, Zabetian Targhi M, Halvaei I, Nosrati R. High-DNA integrity sperm selection using rheotaxis and boundary following behavior in a microfluidic chip. Lab on a Chip. 2023;**23**(9):2241-2248

[85] Ekrami H, Movahedin M, Koosha F, Mazaheri Z, Mokhtari-Dizaji M. The effects of calligonum extract and low-intensity ultrasound on motility, viability, and DNA fragmentation of human frozen-thawed semen samples.

International Journal of Fertility and Sterility. 2020;**14**(2):84-90. DOI: 10.22074/ijfs.2020.5896

[86] Kwizera EA, Sun M, White AM, Li J, He X. Methods of generating dielectrophoretic force for microfluidic manipulation of bioparticles. ACS Biomaterials Science & Engineering. 2021;7(6):2043-2063

[87] Huang HY, Lai YL, Yao DJ. Dielectrophoretic microfluidic device for in vitro fertilization. Micromachines. 2018;**9**(3):135

[88] Kocur OM, Xie P, Cheung S, Souness S, McKnight M, Rosenwaks Z, et al. Can a sperm selection technique improve embryo ploidy? Andrology. 2023;**11**(8):1605-1612

[89] Banti M, Van Zyl E, Kafetzis D. Sperm preparation with microfluidic sperm sorting chip may improve intracytoplasmic sperm injection outcomes compared to density gradient centrifugation. Reproductive Sciences. 2024;**31**:1695-1704

[90] Morishita N, Miura M, Kobayashi Y, Matsunaga R, Maeda T, Ochi M, et al. P-039 male age is associated with sperm DNA integrity: Selection of high DNA integrity sperm by microfluidics sorting is critical to clinical outcomes in older patients. Human Reproduction. 2022;**37**(Suppl. 1):deac107.036

[91] Ozcan P, Takmaz T, Yazici MGK, Alagoz OA, Yesiladali M, Sevket O, et al. Does the use of microfluidic sperm sorting for the sperm selection improve in vitro fertilization success rates in male factor infertility? Journal of Obstetrics and Gynaecology. 2021;**47**(1):382-388

[92] Ferreira Aderaldo J, Da Silva MK, Ferreira Lanza DC. Does microfluidic sperm selection improve clinical pregnancy and miscarriage outcomes in assisted reproductive treatments? A systematic review and meta-analysis. PLoS ONE. 2023;**18**(11):e0292891

[93] Quinn MM, Jalalian L, Ribeiro S, Ona K, Demirci U, Cedars MI, et al. Microfluidic sorting selects sperm for clinical use with reduced DNA damage compared to density gradient centrifugation with swim-up in split semen samples. Human Reproduction. 2018;**33**(8):1388-1393

Chapter 5

# Detection and Clinical Application of Sperm DNA Fragmentation

*Xiaodong Liang*


## Abstract

Sperm DNA fragmentation (SDF) testing has emerged as a crucial tool in the evaluation of male infertility, providing insights beyond conventional semen analysis. SDF refers to the presence of DNA strand breaks in sperm, which can negatively impact fertilization, embryo development, and pregnancy outcomes. Several diagnostic methods, such as the sperm chromatin structure assay (SCSA), terminal deoxynucleotidyl transferase dUTP nick end labeling (TUNEL) assay, and the single-cell gel electrophoresis (comet) assay, are widely used to assess DNA damage in sperm. Clinically, elevated SDF levels are associated with idiopathic infertility, recurrent pregnancy loss, and poor outcomes in assisted reproductive technologies (ART) like in vitro fertilization (IVF) and intracytoplasmic sperm injection (ICSI). SDF testing is gaining importance in guiding therapeutic strategies, including lifestyle interventions, antioxidant therapy, and consideration of advanced ART techniques. Thus, the assessment of sperm DNA integrity plays a vital role in personalized reproductive medicine, optimizing treatment and improving fertility outcomes for couples facing infertility challenges.


**Keywords:** sperm DNA fragmentation, SCSA, TUNEL, SCD, comet, varicocele, unexplained male infertility, early natural miscarriage, in vitro fertilization

## 1. Introduction

Sperm DNA fragmentation is considered a crucial biological marker for male infertility and has gained increasing attention in recent years. It is significant in the evaluation and treatment decision-making for infertility, as well as in prognostic assessments. Due to various factors affecting sperm, unlike somatic cells, sperm lack robust DNA repair capabilities and apoptotic self-cleansing abilities. Therefore, testing for sperm DNA fragmentation is vital. By detecting and assessing the level of sperm DNA fragmentation, potential fertility issues can be identified, guiding personalized treatment and intervention measures, thereby enhancing fertility success rates and male reproductive health.

## 2. Definition of DNA fragmentation

Sperm DNA fragmentation (SDF) refers to the phenomenon of DNA strand breaks or damage in sperm [1]. Typically, healthy sperm DNA should be intact and tightly packed, but in certain conditions, sperm DNA may exhibit breaks or damage, thus affecting its function and quality.

## 3. Causes and mechanisms of DNA fragmentation

The causes of DNA fragmentation include intrinsic factors (susceptibility, compared to somatic cells) (**Figure 1**), and the unique nature of sperm as a type of germ cell. Sperm originate from spermatogonial cells through a two-stage division process to form haploid cells, which undergo DNA replication and chromosome separation, risking DNA strand breaks and damage. Furthermore, after sperm cells are formed, they undergo morphological changes where histones are replaced by protamines, and some organelles are gradually discarded while the residual cytoplasm is concentrated until it disappears. Similar to somatic cells, the factors damaging sperm DNA include both internal factors and exposure to certain external factors. After DNA damage, cells initiate repair mechanisms; when severe DNA damage cannot be repaired, cells activate cleanup mechanisms. However, when these repair and cleanup mechanisms fail, DNA damage will appear in the terminal cells.

### 3.1 Sperm DNA replication and recombination

Sperm are highly specialized cells formed through meiosis from spermatogonial cells, experiencing DNA separation and recombination during two stages of cell division. Despite strict regulation of this process, any errors in replication or separation can lead to DNA damage, thus causing strand breaks and fragmentation [2, 3]. The more divisions a cell undergoes, the higher the likelihood of such occurrences.

### 3.2 Conversion of sperm nuclear proteins

During spermatogenesis within the seminiferous tubules of the testes, sperm undergo stages from primordial germ cells to spermatogonia, primary and secondary spermatocytes, spermatids, and finally to spermatozoa. In the sperm formation stage, sperm cells undergo complex differentiation processes, including nuclear elongation and condensation, acrosome formation, chromatin packaging, and protein transformation [4]. The switch from histones to protamines is a key step in sperm formation,

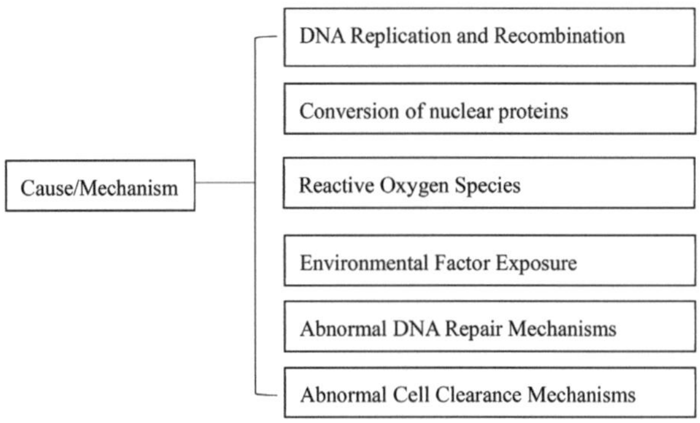


**Figure 1.**
*Cause and mechanism of sperm DNA fragmentation.*

protecting DNA from external damage by tightly packing it, but also making DNA less accessible to repair proteins, thus facilitating DNA fragmentation. Hence, DNA damage repair before this protein transformation is crucial.

### 3.3 Reactive oxygen species

Reactive oxygen species (ROS) can be produced by sperm spontaneously, including hydrogen peroxide ($H_2O_2$) and superoxide anion ($O_2^-$), primarily from normal metabolic activities in mitochondrial respiratory chains and pathways involving nicotinamide adenine dinucleotide phosphate (NADPH) oxidase, xanthine oxidase, and cyclooxygenase [5]. Moderate levels of ROS are involved in physiological processes such as sperm capacitation, acrosome reaction, and flagellar movement [6, 7]. Sperm also possess an antioxidant defense system to neutralize excess ROS and protect cells from oxidative damage, including antioxidant enzymes and antioxidants like vitamin C, vitamin E, coenzyme Q10, and glutathione. These substances can directly neutralize ROS [8]. Normally, the oxidative and antioxidative systems are in dynamic balance. Disruption of this balance can cause various types of damage. Mechanisms of ROS-induced DNA damage include direct damage, where ROS can directly attack DNA molecules, causing base oxidation, deoxyribose oxidation, single-strand breaks, and double-strand breaks. Indirect damage occurs when ROS causes lipid peroxidation of cell membranes, producing peroxidized lipids that further decompose and react with DNA, forming DNA-lipid peroxidation adducts, leading to DNA damage [9]. ROS can also damage DNA repair enzymes, allowing DNA damage to accumulate. High levels of ROS can trigger the release of cytochrome C from mitochondria, activating apoptosis-related proteases like caspase, leading to systemic degradation and fragmentation of DNA.

### 3.4 Environmental factor exposure

Sperm DNA fragmentation can be induced by various environmental factors, each of which contributes to the degradation of sperm DNA integrity in different ways. Common factors include ionizing radiation, elevated temperatures, and a range of environmental pollutants such as heavy metals, pesticides, and industrial chemicals. These elements can cause direct or indirect DNA damage, leading to increased fragmentation and reduced sperm quality, ultimately impacting male fertility. Understanding the specific mechanisms through which these factors contribute to sperm DNA fragmentation is crucial for developing strategies to mitigate their effects.

Ionizing radiation is a potent environmental factor known to cause significant DNA damage. It achieves this through high-energy interactions that directly break the DNA double helix or generate ROS that induce oxidative stress, leading to further DNA damage [10]. Sperm cells, particularly vulnerable due to their limited DNA repair capabilities, are highly susceptible to fragmentation when exposed to ionizing radiation. This exposure disrupts the integrity of the DNA, increasing the incidence of fragmentation and negatively affecting male reproductive health [11].

Exposure to elevated temperatures is another significant cause of sperm DNA fragmentation [12]. High temperatures induce oxidative stress by disrupting cellular metabolism and mitochondrial function, leading to excessive production of ROS [13]. Additionally, heat exposure can compromise the sperm's antioxidant defense mechanisms, exacerbating oxidative damage and resulting in increased DNA fragmentation, thereby reducing the fertilization potential of the sperm.

Environmental pollutants are significant contributors to sperm DNA fragmentation. These pollutants can induce DNA damage through multiple pathways [14]. Heavy metals, for example, can disrupt mitochondrial function, leading to the overproduction of ROS, which damages the DNA [15, 16]. Pesticides and other chemicals may directly cause DNA strand breaks or interfere with enzymes crucial for DNA repair, preventing the correction of damage and increasing fragmentation.

Unhealthy lifestyle choices, such as smoking and excessive alcohol consumption, are also linked to increased sperm DNA fragmentation [17]. Smoking introduces a variety of harmful chemicals, including nicotine and polycyclic aromatic hydrocarbons, which generate ROS and cause oxidative stress, leading to DNA damage in sperm [18]. Alcohol consumption, particularly in excessive amounts, can disrupt the balance of antioxidants and increase oxidative stress [19], similarly contributing to DNA fragmentation. Both smoking and alcohol consumption also impair the body's natural DNA repair mechanisms [20], further exacerbating sperm DNA damage.

Chronic psychological stress is another factor that can lead to sperm DNA fragmentation [21]. Stress activates the hypothalamic-pituitary-adrenal axis, resulting in the release of cortisol and other stress hormones, which can negatively affect spermatogenesis. Additionally, stress can induce oxidative stress, leading to the overproduction of ROS, which damages sperm DNA [22]. Psychological stress may also disrupt the balance of hormones essential for sperm production and maturation, further contributing to DNA fragmentation and reduced sperm quality.

In summary, sperm DNA fragmentation is influenced by a wide range of factors, each of which contributes to DNA damage through mechanisms such as oxidative stress, direct DNA interaction, and impairment of DNA repair processes. Understanding these mechanisms is crucial for developing strategies to minimize exposure and protect male reproductive health.

### 3.5 Medications

Medication-induced sperm DNA damage is common, such as antibiotics and Chemotherapy drugs. Improper or excessive use can also produce side effects on human cells, including affecting sperm DNA structure [23–25]. However, the specific mechanisms of action and drug types may vary among individuals. Male patients undergoing chemotherapy should monitor and protect sperm quality. Therefore, for patients who need long-term medication, regular sperm quality testing is recommended to detect and resolve issues promptly. Avoiding drug abuse and arbitrary changes in medication dosage can help reduce potential risks to sperm quality.

### 3.6 Abnormal DNA repair mechanisms

During spermatogenesis, DNA may suffer various types of damage, including single-strand breaks, double-strand breaks, base modifications, and base mismatches. Different factors produce different types of DNA damage [26], and each type of damage has corresponding repair mechanisms [27]. Sperm are the terminal products of male germ cell development. DNA damage in sperm is relatively difficult to repair due to the high compression of DNA and the transformation of nuclear proteins, which makes repair mechanisms difficult to access and recognize DNA damage. Additionally, mature sperm almost lack cytoplasm, meaning they are deficient in many essential repair proteins and enzymes [28]. Therefore, the special nature of sperm determines that their DNA damage repair capabilities are lower than those of somatic cells, making them more prone to fragmentation. Finally, the polymorphism of repair factors is also associated with sperm DNA damage [29].

### 3.7 Abnormal cell clearance mechanisms

If severe DNA damage cannot be repaired, cells initiate apoptosis to eliminate damaged cells and prevent further harm to the body. The initiation of apoptosis involves the activation and interaction of multiple apoptosis-related proteins, such as the bcl-2 family proteins and Caspase family proteins [30]. Bcl-2 family proteins play a significant role in apoptosis regulation by regulating the permeability of the mitochondrial outer membrane to release apoptosis-inducing factors (such as Cytochrome C), thereby activating the caspase cascade reaction, leading to cell apoptosis. Once the apoptosis program starts, cells undergo a series of morphological and biochemical changes, such as cell shrinkage, nuclear envelope rupture, and DNA fragmentation. Eventually, apoptotic cells are recognized and cleared by surrounding phagocytic cells, thereby maintaining tissue homeostasis and immune balance. In sperm, characteristic events include increased expression density of Fas on the cell surface, activation of nucleases, and externalization of phosphatidylserine on the cell membrane. During spermatogenesis, when DNA is severely damaged or developmentally abnormal, some spermatocytes undergo apoptosis, and their DNA is cut into fragments by nucleases. However, due to various reasons, these fragments are not completely degraded, and the apoptotic process of damaged cells may be interrupted, potentially not being effectively cleared [31, 32]. These cells continue to develop into sperm, resulting in sperm carrying fragmented DNA appearing in semen. It has been observed that infertile males have a higher Fas expression rate in their sperm [33].

Therefore, some believe that this abnormal programmed cell death in reproductive cells may be cleared through natural selection processes, rather than in the traditional form of being engulfed by phagocytic cells [34].

## 4. Detection of DNA fragmentation

Sperm DNA fragmentation is commonly assessed using several methods (**Figure 2**), each with distinct features. The sperm chromatin structure assay (SCSA)

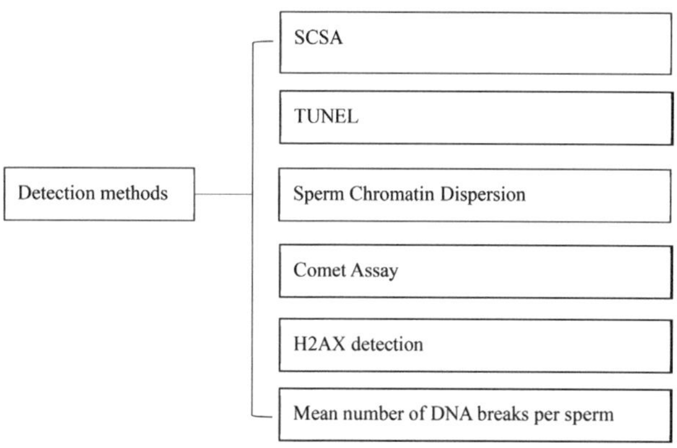


**Figure 2.**
*Detection methods of Sperm DNA fragmentation.*

measures DNA denaturation susceptibility, while the Terminal deoxynucleotidyl transferase dUTP Nick End Labeling (TUNEL) assay directly labels DNA breaks. The comet assay visualizes DNA damage via gel electrophoresis, allowing for single-cell analysis. Each of these methods varies in sensitivity and clinical utility. Emerging techniques, such as γH2AX detection, identify DNA damage through histone modification, offering a more detailed understanding of chromatin integrity. Additionally, measuring the average number of DNA breaks per sperm provides a refined metric for assessing sperm quality.

### 4.1 Terminal deoxynucleotidyl transferase dUTP Nick end labeling

The Terminal deoxynucleotidyl transferase dUTP Nick End Labeling (TUNEL) method uses terminal deoxynucleotidyl transferase (TdT) to recognize a large number of 3'-OH ends exposed during cell apoptosis or DNA damage and add dUTP to the ends, labeling dUTP with fluorescence. This allows the 3'-OH ends to be marked with fluorescent signals, which can be detected by fluorescence microscopy or flow cytometry [35]. By measuring the fluorescence signal intensity, the presence of DNA fragmentation can be assessed. The TUNEL method, being a direct detection method for DNA breaks, has high sensitivity and specificity. It allows for quantitative assessment through image analysis under a microscope or flow cytometry. However, this method has a high false-positive rate and requires skilled operators. Correct operation and appropriate control experiments are crucial for accurate results.

### 4.2 Sperm chromatin structure assay

The Sperm Chromatin Structure Assay (SCSA) is another technique for assessing sperm DNA fragmentation and chromatin structure integrity. It involves treating sperm samples with an acidic solution, causing chromatin destabilization and partial unwinding, thus exposing DNA breaks. Under the influence of acridine orange, double-stranded DNA emits green fluorescence, while single-stranded DNA emits red fluorescence [36]. By measuring the ratio of double-stranded DNA (green fluorescence) to single-stranded DNA (red fluorescence) using flow cytometry, the DNA Fragmentation Index (DFI) results can be obtained. The SCSA method has high sensitivity and specificity, accurately detecting sperm DNA fragmentation and chromatin destabilization. It requires flow cytometry equipment and skilled technical operation. Standardization of sample processing, staining, and flow cytometry analysis is crucial for accurate results. Flow cytometers provide quantitative results with good repeatability and comparability, making this method widely used in clinical and research settings [37]. Results can be compared between different laboratories.

### 4.3 Sperm chromatin dispersion

The Sperm Chromatin Dispersion (SCD) method is a technique for assessing sperm DNA fragmentation by observing the dispersion patterns of sperm chromatin after specific treatments. It involves removing nuclear proteins from sperm using strong alkaline or proteolytic solutions. Normal sperm chromatin forms large and uniform dispersion rings (halos), while sperm with DNA fragmentation forms smaller or no dispersion rings. After staining, sperm chromatin dispersion patterns can be observed and analyzed under a microscope. By analyzing these patterns, the degree of DNA fragmentation can be assessed [38]. The SCD method has high sensitivity and specificity, effectively distinguishing normal chromatin structure from DNA-fragmented chromatin. It is relatively simple and does not require complex equipment [39]. It can quantitatively provide the percentage of fragmented sperm, offering good repeatability. However, due to its reliance on manual observation, it may have some subjectivity. The SCD method can only detect total DNA damage, with advancements in technology, recent studies have developed a new, rapid technique based on single-strand breaks for detecting double-strand DNA damage [40].

### 4.4 Comet assay

The Comet Assay is a test that detects damaged DNA through electrophoresis. After releasing sperm DNA, it undergoes electrophoresis under alkaline (or neutral) conditions. Damaged DNA migrates out of the cell nucleus under the influence of the electric field, forming a "comet" shape. The more DNA fragments in the tail, the more severe the DNA damage [41, 42]. The Comet Assay has high sensitivity and can detect low levels of DNA damage, including single-strand breaks, double-strand breaks, and alkaline-labile sites. It is applicable to various cell types and different types of DNA damage, providing detailed quantitative data to assess DNA damage. However, the technique requires high expertise, and image analysis may have some subjectivity. It requires experienced operators to optimize electrophoresis conditions and staining procedures to ensure accurate results [43]. In recent years, researchers have designed the bidirectional Comet Assay, based on the same principle but conducting electrophoresis under alkaline and neutral conditions on the same agarose gel but in XY directions [44]. This produces different comet images, and image analysis software can analyze the tailing conditions in both directions to determine whether the DNA damage is mainly single-strand or double-strand breaks.

### 4.5 Other methods

With the development of testing technology in recent years, some new methods for detecting sperm DNA fragmentation have emerged. Yan and others introduced a new method that can quantitatively detect the number of DNA breaks per sperm, accurately reflecting the extent of DNA damage. They use terminal deoxynucleotidyl transferase to recognize DNA breaks producing 3'-OH and catalyze its polymerization with dATP, generating extended poly(A) tails. Fluorescent group 6-carboxyfluorescein (FAM) and fluorescence quencher 1 (BHQ-1) labeled probes poly(T) are then used to match the extended poly(A) tails. After nuclease IV hydrolyzes the bound probe, the fluorescent group FAM loses the quenching effect of the quencher and emits fluorescence. After this process, new probes can continue to bind to poly-A, producing secondary amplification. Each breakpoint in sperm DNA follows the described process, making the increase in fluorescence rate proportional to the number of breakpoints in sperm DNA. The fluorescence increase in sperm DNA samples after the reaction can be used to calculate the number of terminal sites in sperm DNA samples, converting it into the average number of DNA strand breaks for quantitative assessment of sperm DNA fragmentation [45, 46]. This method correlates well with SCSA testing results and distinguishes semen quality with a good area under the ROC curve, promising to become a new technology for future detection.

Detection of sperm DNA damage using the histone H2AX detection method is another important technical approach. Specifically, it involves detecting phosphorylated H2AX (γ-H2AX) to assess the extent of sperm DNA damage. γ-H2AX is a marker of DNA damage, especially double-strand breaks, and its physiological role is to rapidly recruit DNA repair and apoptosis proteins to the site of damage to participate in the DNA repair process [47]. Specific methods for H2AX detection include immunofluorescence, which is one of the common methods for detecting γ-H2AX. By binding a specific antibody to γ-H2AX and using a fluorescent dye to label the antibody, the fluorescence signal in the sperm cell nucleus can be observed under a fluorescence microscope. When sperm DNA is damaged, the content of γ-H2AX increases, producing a strong fluorescence signal in the cell nucleus [48].

Flow cytometry: Flow cytometry can also be used to detect γ-H2AX levels in sperm. By rapidly and extensively analyzing sperm cells using a flow cytometer, the γ-H2AX content in each sperm cell can be accurately measured, thereby assessing the extent of sperm DNA damage [49].

Western blotting: Additionally, Western blotting is another common detection method. By extracting protein samples from sperm cells and binding a specific antibody to γ-H2AX, the presence and content of γ-H2AX can be detected during gel electrophoresis and blotting processes [50]. The level of γ-H2AX can reflect the extent of sperm DNA damage, making the H2AX detection method useful for assessing sperm quality. High levels of γ-H2AX may indicate significant sperm DNA damage, potentially affecting fertilization and embryo development processes [48].

Researching the mechanisms of sperm DNA damage: Through the H2AX detection method, researchers can further explore the mechanisms of sperm DNA damage, providing a theoretical basis for developing new treatment methods and prevention measures.

## 5. Clinical applications of DNA fragmentation testing

SDF testing has significant clinical applications in male fertility assessment (**Figure 3**). It helps analyze the impact of varicocele on sperm, identify underlying causes of infertility that conventional semen analysis might miss, and offer deeper insights into sperm quality. In cases of recurrent pregnancy loss (RPL), SDF testing is valuable in determining potential male factors contributing to miscarriages. Additionally, it is used to predict outcomes in assisted reproductive technologies (ART), such as in vitro fertilization (IVF) and intracytoplasmic sperm injection (ICSI), where high DNA fragmentation is associated with lower success rates. Overall, SDF testing plays a crucial role in diagnosing male infertility and optimizing fertility treatments.

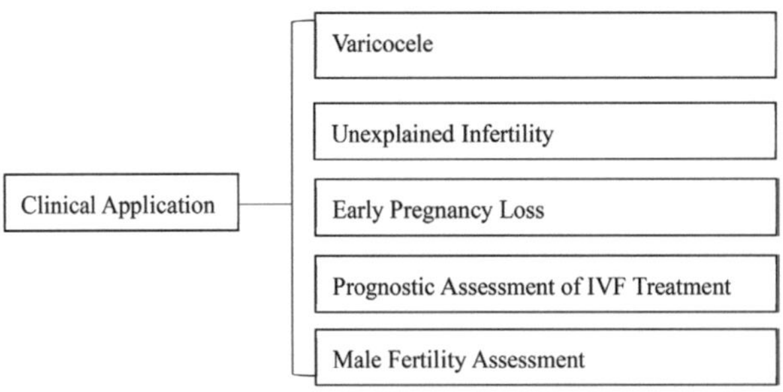


**Figure 3.**
*Clinical application of sperm DNA fragmentation.*

### 5.1 Varicocele

Varicocele refers to a series of symptoms caused by abnormal, tortuous dilation or elongation of the pampiniform venous plexus within the spermatic cord, a common disease in the male urogenital system [51]. Its main symptoms include scrotal pain, discomfort, or dampness when sitting or standing for extended periods, and it may lead to a continuous decline in semen quality and even testicular atrophy, making it a common cause of male infertility. Venous blood stasis can increase scrotal temperature, increase the production of ROS, and reduce the levels of antioxidants, thereby damaging the integrity of sperm DNA [52–54]. Therefore, assessing sperm DNA fragmentation in varicocele patients can help understand the extent of DNA damage caused by blood stasis, aiding early diagnosis and assessing the impact of varicocele on fertility. Compared to traditional semen analysis, sperm DNA fragmentation testing can more sensitively detect sperm damage that traditional analysis might miss [55]. Additionally, it can help evaluate the recovery of fertility after varicocele surgery [56].

### 5.2 Unexplained infertility

Unexplained infertility refers to infertility that remains undiagnosed after a comprehensive reproductive health examination. In such cases, traditional semen analysis (including sperm count, motility, and morphology) may appear normal, but the couple may still have difficulty conceiving naturally. Studies have shown that sperm DNA fragmentation may be present in these couples, making sperm DNA fragmentation testing a supplementary diagnostic tool for unexplained infertility [57]. It provides additional information on sperm quality, helping identify potential fertility issues.

### 5.3 Early pregnancy loss

Early Pregnancy Loss (EPL) typically refers to natural miscarriages or embryonic arrest that occur during the early stages of pregnancy, specifically before the 20th week of gestation. At this stage, the embryo or fetus fails to continue normal development for various reasons and is spontaneously expelled from the body, resulting in the termination of the pregnancy. The causes of EPL are complex and varied, including genetic factors, immunological abnormalities, infections, uterine anatomical defects, endocrine disorders, thrombosis, and more. Genetic factors are considered the primary cause of pregnancy loss due to chromosomal abnormalities in the embryo [58], accounting for 50–60% of all miscarriage cases. Since embryonic genetic information comes from both parents, sperm factors, particularly sperm DNA fragmentation, have increasingly gained attention in recent years [59, 60]. For fertilized oocytes, sperm DNA damage present in the maternal cell does not manifest during the early zygotic stage under the dominance of maternal genes [61]. As the embryo develops, embryonic genes begin to activate and express, a process known as "maternal to zygotic transition" [62], when the impact of sperm factors begins to emerge. The oocyte has limited DNA repair capabilities [63], relying on intracellular repair factors for limited repair. Unrepairable DNA damage becomes very apparent after embryo implantation, leading to abnormalities in embryo development, such as cell degeneration, genetic mutations, and developmental arrest, thereby increasing the risk of miscarriage and pregnancy loss [64]. Therefore, the impact of sperm factors on the embryo usually manifests later in embryonic development, known as "late paternal effects." However, there is still controversy regarding these studies.

For such patients, sperm DNA fragmentation testing can be part of the assessment, helping identify potential male factors.

### 5.4 Prognostic assessment in In vitro fertilization treatment

Sperm DNA fragmentation plays a significant role in the prognostic assessment of IVF and ICSI. High levels of sperm DNA fragmentation may affect sperm fertilization capability. Studies have shown that men with high levels of sperm DNA fragmentation have lower fertilization rates in IVF or ICSI [65–67]. Subsequently, this leads to chromosomal abnormalities or developmental disorders in embryos [68], thereby increasing the miscarriage rate and ultimately affecting pregnancy outcomes, including clinical pregnancy rates and live birth rates. By testing and assessing sperm DNA fragmentation levels, potential fertility issues can be identified, and personalized treatment and intervention can be implemented to reduce sperm DNA fragmentation levels or select sperm with higher DNA integrity in the IVF lab [69]. Optimizing assisted reproductive technology can help improve fertilization rates, embryo quality, and pregnancy success rates while reducing miscarriage risks.

The IVF process involves fertilization, cleavage, early embryo, and blastocyst formation. The impact of sperm DNA fragmentation on IVF fertilization outcomes has been widely reported in the literature, but the results are inconsistent. A systematic review analysis suggests that in conventional IVF, which primarily uses droplet culture for fertilization, sperm DNA fragmentation reduces the fertilization rate of conventional IVF because it undergoes a sperm selection process where sperm with DNA fragmentation cannot adhere to the zona pellucida of the oocyte. In contrast, sperm used in ICSI undergo manual selection, typically selecting sperm with normal morphology and strong motility, making the impact of sperm DNA fragmentation on ICSI fertilization rates unclear [70]. Additionally, the heterogeneity of fertilization outcomes in ICSI mentioned in this systematic review may be related to the strong subjectivity involved in technician-selected sperm. The mechanism may involve factors associated with DNA damage, such as ROS, simultaneously destroying proteins related to fertilization function, causing abnormal protein expression, and preventing adhesion to and fusion with the oocyte membrane. Further research is needed to understand these mechanisms.

Sperm DNA fragmentation may cause genetic material abnormalities, affecting embryo development. Therefore, it may impact the quality of early-stage IVF embryos. Although many studies have reported the impact of DNA fragmentation on embryo quality [71], the conclusions are also inconsistent. A systematic review study indicates that sperm with double-strand DNA damage have the most significant impact on embryo quality, and among the tests, the Comet assay can detect double-strand DNA damage, thus providing strong predictive power for embryo quality [72]. As the embryo development process proceeds post-IVF, the embryonic genome begins to express, marking the start of the maternal-to-zygotic transition effect and the emergence of paternal effects [61]. The impact of sperm factors on the embryo begins to manifest. However, there is no consensus on the earliest stage when paternal effects first appear. Some believe that it starts after embryo implantation, leading to early miscarriages due to abnormal genetic material. Others believe that it starts from Day 5 post-fertilization, manifested as a reduced blastocyst formation rate [65, 73]. Still, others believe that it begins from the early embryo stage, manifested as a reduced availability of embryos on Day 3 post-fertilization [74].

The clinical pregnancy rate during the transfer cycle is an important outcome measure for the success of in vitro fertilization-embryo transfer (IVF-ET). Most studies suggest that sperm DNA fragmentation has a negative impact on the clinical pregnancy rate. A systematic review study indicates that regardless of the detection method used for sperm DNA fragmentation and the fertilization method used, the detection results have a negative impact on the clinical pregnancy rate [70]. Among these, TUNEL and Comet are strongly correlated with pregnancy outcomes. However, some meta-analyses conclude that sperm DNA fragmentation is not related to the clinical pregnancy rate [75]. This may be because these analyses did not exclude factors such as advanced maternal age and female factors causing infertility. Once such factors are excluded, the significance of the differences in predicted outcomes increases markedly [70, 76].

The cumulative live birth rate is another important clinical outcome measure for IVF-ET success. It considers a complete treatment set, where embryos obtained from one oocyte retrieval are transferred multiple times until all embryos are transferred or a live birth occurs [77]. The percentage of treatment sets with a live birth record among all treatment sets is the cumulative live birth rate per oocyte retrieval cycle. As embryo transfer includes both fresh and frozen embryo transfers, the cumulative live birth rate is considered a more comprehensive measure of IVF success. Research on the impact of sperm DNA fragmentation on the cumulative live birth rate per oocyte retrieval cycle is a relatively new field, and to date, only a few studies exist. Among them, Vončina and others found that sperm DNA fragmentation significantly reduces the cumulative live birth rate per oocyte retrieval cycle [78]. Conversely, Liang and colleagues further analyzed and found that a reduction in the number of embryos, leading to fewer transfer opportunities, may be the reason. Based on this, they propose that the number of embryos could be considered a predictive tool to analyze in advance the impact of DNA fragmentation on the cumulative live birth rate [79].

### 5.5 Male fertility assessment

Sperm DNA damage is inversely related to the chances of natural conception. When the SDF index, as measured by SCSA, falls within the 20–30% range, the likelihood of achieving a natural pregnancy diminishes [80]. Additionally, some studies indicate that SDF levels exceeding 30% are linked to lower pregnancy rates [81, 82] and longer times to conceive [20].

As previously mentioned, external factors causing sperm DNA damage include environmental factors and medication factors. Testing for DNA fragmentation can assess the extent of damage caused by the environment (including radiation, high temperatures, chemicals, etc.) and certain medications (such as antibiotics, antitumor drugs, etc.) on sperm DNA, indirectly reflecting the impact on male fertility [83]. Additionally, conducting sperm DNA fragmentation testing before planning for childbirth can assess the reproductive health status of men, identify potential fertility issues [84], and take preventive measures against infertility. Therefore, sperm DNA fragmentation holds significant importance in the assessment of male fertility [85].

## 6. Conclusion

Sperm DNA fragmentation is an important biological marker for male infertility and miscarriage, with causes including intrinsic physiological processes, susceptibility risks, and external environmental factors. Various detection methods provide sensitive means to assess the extent of DNA fragmentation, helping reveal issues with sperm quality. As new detection methods emerge, more sensitive, accurate, and specific diagnostic technologies continue to enrich and improve. In clinical practice, testing for sperm DNA fragmentation not only aids in diagnosing and assessing fertility-related diseases but also guides the optimization of in vitro fertilization techniques and the assessment of male reproductive health. The advancements in these studies and technologies provide important tools and ideas for enhancing male fertility and the success rate of assisted reproductive technologies.

## Acknowledgements

The author thanks all individuals who contributed to this article.

## Conflict of interest

The author declares no competing interests.

## Author details

Xiaodong Liang
Clinical Transformation and Application Key Lab for Obstetrics and Gynecology, Pediatrics, and Reproductive Medicine of Jiangmen, Jiangmen, China

*Address all correspondence to: 229290147@qq.com

## References

[1] Qiu Y, Yang H, Li C. Progress in research on sperm DNA fragmentation. Medical Science Monitor. 2020;**26**: e918746. DOI: 10.12659/MSM.918746

[2] Xie C, Wang W, Tu C. Meiotic recombination: Insights into its mechanisms and its role in human reproduction with a special focus on non-obstructive azoospermia. Human Reproduction Update. 2022;**28**:763-797. DOI: 10.1093/humupd/dmac024

[3] Tempest HG. Meiotic recombination errors, the origin of sperm aneuploidy and clinical recommendations. Systems Biology in Reproductive Medicine. 2011;**57**:93-101. DOI: 10.3109/19396368.2010.504879

[4] Leduc F, Nkoma GB, Boissonneault G. Spermiogenesis and DNA repair: A possible etiology of human infertility and genetic disorders. Systems Biology in Reproductive Medicine. 2008;**54**:3-10. DOI: 10.1080/19396360701876823

[5] Gibb Z, Griffin RA, Aitken RJ. Functions and effects of reactive oxygen species in male fertility. Animal Reproduction Science. 2020;**220**:106456. DOI: 10.1016/j.anireprosci.2020.106456

[6] Chianese R, Pierantoni R. Mitochondrial reactive oxygen species (ROS) production alters sperm quality. Antioxidants. 2021;**10**:92. DOI: 10.3390/antiox10010092

[7] O'Flaherty C. Redox regulation of mammalian sperm capacitation. Asian Journal of Andrology. 2015;**17**:583-590. DOI: 10.4103/1008-682X.153303

[8] O'Flaherty C, Scarlata E. Oxidative stress and reproductive function: The protection of mammalian spermatozoa against oxidative stress. Reproduction. 2022;**164**:F67-F78. DOI: 10.1530/REP-22-0200

[9] Aitken RJ, Gibb Z, Baker MA. Causes and consequences of oxidative stress in spermatozoa. Reproduction Fertility and Development. 2016;**28**:1-10. DOI: 10.1071/RD15325

[10] Kumar D, Salian SR, Kalthur G. Semen abnormalities, sperm DNA damage and global hypermethylation in health workers occupationally exposed to ionizing radiation. PLoS One. 2013;**8**:e69927. DOI: 10.1371/journal.pone.0069927

[11] Fuller N, Smith JT, Ford AT. Impacts of ionising radiation on sperm quality, DNA integrity and post-fertilisation development in marine and freshwater crustaceans. Ecotoxicology and Environmental Safety. 2019;**186**:109764. DOI: 10.1016/j.ecoenv.2019.109764

[12] Durairajanayagam D, Agarwal A, Ong C. Causes, effects and molecular mechanisms of testicular heat stress. Reproductive Biomedicine Online. 2015;**30**:14-27. DOI: 10.1016/j.rbmo.2014.09.018

[13] Zhao F, Whiting S, Lambourne S. Melatonin alleviates heat stress-induced oxidative stress and apoptosis in human spermatozoa. Free Radical Biology and Medicine. 2021;**164**:410-416. DOI: 10.1016/j.freeradbiomed.2021.01.014

[14] Marinaro C, Lettieri G, Chianese T. Exploring the molecular and toxicological mechanism associated with interactions between heavy metals and the reproductive system of Mytilus galloprovincialis. Comparative

Biochemistry and Physiology C-Toxicology & Pharmacology. 2024;**275**:109778. DOI: 10.1016/j.cbpc.2023.109778

[15] Zhou Y, Fu XM, He DL. Evaluation of urinary metal concentrations and sperm DNA damage in infertile men from an infertility clinic. Environmental Toxicology and Pharmacology. 2016;**45**:68-73. DOI: 10.1016/j.etap.2016.05.020

[16] Saberi E, Mohammadrezaei FM, Jazayeri O. Astaxanthin induces the expression of CatSper1 gene and Protects sperms in toxicity induced by cadmium in mice. Drug Research. 2021;**71**:512-519. DOI: 10.1055/a-1553-3265

[17] Szabó A, Váncsa S, Hegyi P. Lifestyle-, environmental-, and additional health factors associated with an increased sperm DNA fragmentation: A systematic review and meta-analysis. Reproductive Biology and Endocrinology. 2023;**21**:5. DOI: 10.1186/s12958-023-01054-0

[18] Osadchuk L, Kleshchev M, Osadchuk A. Effects of cigarette smoking on semen quality, reproductive hormone levels, metabolic profile, zinc and sperm DNA fragmentation in men: Results from a population-based study. Frontiers in Endocrinology. 2023;**14**:1255304. DOI: 10.3389/fendo.2023.1255304

[19] Nguyen-Thanh T, Hoang-Thi AP, Anh TD. Investigating the association between alcohol intake and male reproductive function: A current meta-analysis. Heliyon. 2023;**9**:e15723. DOI: 10.1016/j.heliyon.2023.e15723

[20] Amor H, Hammadeh ME, Mohd I. Impact of heavy alcohol consumption and cigarette smoking on sperm DNA integrity. Andrologia. 2022;**54**:e14434. DOI: 10.1111/and.14434

[21] Abdollahi F, Farhang DS, Amanpour S. Effect of Co-exposure to heat and psychological stressors on sperm DNA and semen parameters. Toxicology Reports. 2021;**8**:1948-1954. DOI: 10.1016/j.toxrep.2021.11.015

[22] Jiang Y, Botchway B, Hu Z. Overexpression of SIRT1 inhibits corticosterone-induced autophagy. Neuroscience. 2019;**411**:11-22. DOI: 10.1016/j.neuroscience.2019.05.035

[23] Tímermans A, Vázquez R, Otero F. Antibiotic toxicity on human spermatozoa assessed using the sperm DNA fragmentation dynamic assay. Andrologia. 2022;**54**:e14328. DOI: 10.1111/and.14328

[24] Morris ID. Sperm DNA damage and cancer treatment. International Journal of Andrology. 2002;**25**:255-261. DOI: 10.1046/j.1365-2605.2002.00372.x

[25] Pecou S, Moinard N, Walschaerts M. Ribavirin and pegylated interferon treatment for hepatitis C was associated not only with semen alterations but also with sperm deoxyribonucleic acid fragmentation in humans. Fertility and Sterility. 2009;**91**:917-933. DOI: 10.1016/j.fertnstert.2008.07.1755

[26] Hourcade JD, Perez-Crespo M, Fernandez-Gonzalez R. Selection against spermatozoa with fragmented DNA after postovulatory mating depends on the type of damage. Reproductive Biology and Endocrinology. 2010;**8**:9. DOI: 10.1186/1477-7827-8-9

[27] Wan W, Zhang C, Zhang Q. Exploring the mechanisms of Yishen Tongluo decoction on repairing DNA damage in mouse Spermatogonia cells based on whole transcriptome sequencing. American Journal of Mens Health. 2024;**18**:1044156604. DOI: 10.1177/15579883241246908

[28] De Iuliis GN, Newey RJ, King BV. Mobile phone radiation induces reactive oxygen species production and DNA damage in human spermatozoa in vitro. PLoS One. 2009;**4**:e6446. DOI: 10.1371/journal.pone.0006446

[29] Gu A, Ji G, Zhou Y. Polymorphisms of nucleotide-excision repair genes may contribute to sperm DNA fragmentation and male infertility. Reproductive Biomedicine Online. 2010;**21**:602-609. DOI: 10.1016/j.rbmo.2010.06.025

[30] Zhu G, Zhang Y, Dong J. Association between body mass index and male sperm apoptosis and apoptosis-related factors. Diabetes Metabolic Syndrome and Obesity-Targets and Therapy. 2021;**14**:1043-1051. DOI: 10.2147/DMSO.S289923

[31] Libman J, Gabriel MS, Sairam MR. Catalase can protect spermatozoa of FSH receptor knock-out mice against oxidant-induced DNA damage in vitro. International Journal of Andrology. 2010;**33**:818-822. DOI: 10.1111/j.1365-2605.2009.01032.x

[32] Kuchakulla M, Narasimman M, Khodamoradi K. How defective spermatogenesis affects sperm DNA integrity. Andrologia. 2021;**53**:e13615. DOI: 10.1111/and.13615

[33] McVicar CM, McClure N, Williamson K. Incidence of Fas positivity and deoxyribonucleic acid double-stranded breaks in human ejaculated sperm. Fertility and Sterility. 2004;**81**(Suppl 1):767-774. DOI: 10.1016/j.fertnstert.2003.10.013

[34] Sakkas D, Mariethoz E, St JJ. Abnormal sperm parameters in humans are indicative of an abortive apoptotic mechanism linked to the Fas-mediated pathway. Experimental Cell Research. 1999;**251**:350-355. DOI: 10.1006/excr.1999.4586

[35] Sharma R, Iovine C, Agarwal A. TUNEL assay-standardized method for testing sperm DNA fragmentation. Andrologia. 2021;**53**:e13738. DOI: 10.1111/and.13738

[36] Henkel R, Hoogendijk CF, Bouic PJ. TUNEL assay and SCSA determine different aspects of sperm DNA damage. Andrologia. 2010;**42**:305-313. DOI: 10.1111/j.1439-0272.2009.01002.x

[37] Yuan M, Huang L, Leung WT. Sperm DNA fragmentation valued by SCSA and its correlation with conventional sperm parameters in male partner of recurrent spontaneous abortion couple. BioScience Trends. 2019;**13**:152-159. DOI: 10.5582/bst.2018.01292

[38] Sivanarayana T, Ravi KC, Jaya PG. Sperm DNA fragmentation assay by sperm chromatin dispersion (SCD): Correlation between DNA fragmentation and outcome of intracytoplasmic sperm injection. Reproductive Medicine and Biology. 2014;**13**:87-94. DOI: 10.1007/s12522-013-0168-7

[39] Unsal E, Turan V, Aktuna S. Effects of pentoxifylline and platelet activating factor on sperm DNA damage. European Journal of Obstetrics & Gynecology and Reproductive Biology. 2016;**197**:125-129. DOI: 10.1016/j.ejogrb.2015.12.016

[40] Wang TE, Lee CI, Huang CC. Innovative technology for evaluation of sperm DNA double-strand breaks diagnoses male factor infertility and prevents reproductive failures. Scientific Reports. 2023;**13**:18996. DOI: 10.1038/s41598-023-46049-4

[41] Pastuszek E, Kiewisz J, Skowronska P. An investigation of the potential effect of sperm nuclear vacuoles in human spermatozoa on DNA fragmentation using a neutral and alkaline comet assay. Andrology. 2017;**5**:392-398. DOI: 10.1111/andr.12324

[42] Ribas-Maynou J, Fernández-Encinas A, García-Peiró A. Human semen cryopreservation: A sperm DNA fragmentation study with alkaline and neutral comet assay. Andrology. 2014;**2**:83-87. DOI: 10.1111/j.2047-2927.2013.00158.x

[43] Ribas-Maynou J, García-Peiró A, Fernandez-Encinas A. Double stranded sperm DNA breaks, measured by comet assay, are associated with unexplained recurrent miscarriage in couples without a female factor. PLoS One. 2012;**7**:e44679. DOI: 10.1371/journal.pone.0044679

[44] Pérez-Llano B, López-Fernández C, García-Casado P. Dynamics of sperm DNA fragmentation in the swine: Ejaculate and temperature effects. Animal Reproduction Science. 2010;**119**:235-243. DOI: 10.1016/j.anireprosci.2010.01.002

[45] Yan B, Ye W, Wang J. Evaluation of sperm DNA integrity by mean number of sperm DNA breaks rather than sperm DNA fragmentation index. Clinical Chemistry. 2022;**68**:540-549. DOI: 10.1093/clinchem/hvab280

[46] Zhou W, Zhang J, Cheng Z. Mean number of DNA breakpoints: Illuminating sperm DNA integrity and in vitro fertilization outcomes. Fertility and Sterility. 2024;**121**:264-270. DOI: 10.1016/j.fertnstert.2023.11.026

[47] Kuo LJ, Yang LX. Gamma-H2AX—A novel biomarker for DNA double-strand breaks. In Vivo. 2008;**22**:305-309

[48] Coban O, Serdarogullari M, Yarkiner Z. Investigating the level of DNA double-strand break in human spermatozoa and its relation to semen characteristics and IVF outcome using phospho-histone H2AX antibody as a biomarker. Andrology. 2020;**8**:421-426. DOI: 10.1111/andr.12689

[49] Zhong HZ, Lv FT, Deng XL. Evaluating γH2AX in spermatozoa from male infertility patients. Fertility and Sterility. 2015;**104**:574-581. DOI: 10.1016/j.fertnstert.2015.06.004

[50] Park HJ, Lee WY, Zhang M. Evaluation of Resmethrin toxicity to neonatal testes in organ culture. Toxicological Sciences. 2020;**173**:53-64. DOI: 10.1093/toxsci/kfz212

[51] Shenoy N, Bhagat TD, Cheville J. Ascorbic acid-induced TET activation mitigates adverse hydroxymethylcytosine loss in renal cell carcinoma. Journal of Clinical Investigation. 2019;**129**:1612-1625. DOI: 10.1172/JCI98747

[52] Agarwal A, Sharma R, Samanta L. Proteomic signatures of infertile men with clinical varicocele and their validation studies reveal mitochondrial dysfunction leading to infertility. Asian Journal of Andrology. 2016;**18**:282-291. DOI: 10.4103/1008-682X.170445

[53] Kamal HM, El-Fallah AA, Abdelbaki SA. Association between seminal granulysin and malondialdehyde in infertile men with varicocele and the potential effect of varicocelectomy. Andrologia. 2020;**52**:e13579. DOI: 10.1111/and.13579

[54] Neto LFT, Campos LR, Roque M. From pathophysiology to practice: Addressing oxidative stress and sperm DNA fragmentation in Varicocele-affected subfertile men. Sociedade Brasileira de. Urologia. 2024;**50**: 530-560. DOI: 10.1590/S1677-5538.IBJU.2024.9917

[55] Jeremias JT, Belardin LB, Okada FK. Oxidative origin of sperm DNA fragmentation in the adult varicocele. International Brazilian Journal of Urology. 2021;**47**:275-283. DOI: 10.1590/S1677-5538.IBJU.2019.0827

[56] Gabriel MS, Chan SW, Alhathal N. Influence of microsurgical varicocelectomy on human sperm mitochondrial DNA copy number: A pilot study. Journal of Assisted Reproduction and Genetics. 2012;**29**:759-764. DOI: 10.1007/s10815-012-9785-z

[57] Agarwal A, Parekh N, Panner SM. Male oxidative stress infertility (MOSI): Proposed terminology and clinical practice guidelines for Management of Idiopathic Male Infertility. World Journal of Mens Health. 2019;**37**:296-312. DOI: 10.5534/wjmh.190055

[58] Dong Y, Li LL, Wang RX. Reproductive outcomes in recurrent pregnancy loss associated with a parental carrier of chromosome abnormalities or polymorphisms. Genetics and Molecular Research. 2014;**13**:2849-2856. DOI: 10.4238/2014.January.17.4

[59] Tan J, Taskin O, Albert A. Association between sperm DNA fragmentation and idiopathic recurrent pregnancy loss: A systematic review and meta-analysis. Reproductive Biomedicine Online. 2019;**38**:951-960. DOI: 10.1016/j.rbmo.2018.12.029

[60] McQueen DB, Zhang J, Robins JC. Sperm DNA fragmentation and recurrent pregnancy loss: A systematic review and meta-analysis. Fertility and Sterility. 2019;**112**:54-60.e3. DOI: 10.1016/j.fertnstert.2019.03.003

[61] Tesarik J, Greco E, Mendoza C. Late, but not early, paternal effect on human embryo development is related to sperm DNA fragmentation. Human Reproduction. 2004;**19**:611-615. DOI: 10.1093/humrep/deh127

[62] Lee MT, Bonneau AR, Giraldez AJ. Zygotic genome activation during the maternal-to-zygotic transition. Annual Review of Cell and Developmental Biology. 2014;**30**:581-613. DOI: 10.1146/annurev-cellbio-100913-013027

[63] Setti AS, Braga D, Provenza RR. Oocyte ability to repair sperm DNA fragmentation: The impact of maternal age on intracytoplasmic sperm injection outcomes. Fertility and Sterility. 2021;**116**:123-129. DOI: 10.1016/j.fertnstert.2020.10.045

[64] Marinaro JA. Sperm DNA fragmentation and its interaction with female factors. Fertility and Sterility. 2023;**120**:715-719. DOI: 10.1016/j.fertnstert.2023.06.001

[65] Wang S, Tan W, Huang Y. Sperm DNA fragmentation measured by sperm chromatin dispersion impacts morphokinetic parameters, fertilization rate and blastocyst quality in ICSI treatments. Zygote. 2022;**30**:72-79. DOI: 10.1017/S0967199421000332

[66] Tang L, Rao M, Yang W. Predictive value of the sperm DNA fragmentation index for low or failed IVF fertilization in men with mild-to-moderate asthenozoospermia. Journal of Gynecology Obstetrics and Human Reproduction. 2021;**50**:101868. DOI: 10.1016/j.jogoh.2020.101868

[67] Ribas-Maynou J, Yeste M, Becerra-Tomás N. Clinical implications of sperm DNA damage in IVF and ICSI: Updated systematic review and meta-analysis. Biological Reviews. 2021;**96**:1284-1300. DOI: 10.1111/brv.12700

[68] Fu W, Cui Q, Yang Z. High sperm DNA fragmentation increased embryo aneuploidy rate in patients undergoing preimplantation genetic testing. Reproductive Biomedicine Online. 2023;**47**:103366. DOI: 10.1016/j.rbmo.2023.103366

[69] Pregl BB, Kovačič B, Vlaisavljević V. Are sperm DNA fragmentation,

hyperactivation, and hyaluronan-binding ability predictive for fertilization and embryo development in in vitro fertilization and intracytoplasmic sperm injection? Fertility and Sterility. 2013;**99**:1233-1241. DOI: 10.1016/j.fertnstert.2012.11.048

[70] Simon L, Emery BR, Carrell DT. Review: Diagnosis and impact of sperm DNA alterations in assisted reproduction. Best Practice & Research Clinical Obstetrics & Gynaecology. 2017;**44**:38-56. DOI: 10.1016/j.bpobgyn.2017.07.003

[71] Vallet-Buisan M, Mecca R, Jones C. Contribution of semen to early embryo development: Fertilization and beyond. Human Reproduction Update. 2023;**29**:395-433. DOI: 10.1093/humupd/dmad006

[72] Ribas-Maynou J, Benet J. Single and double Strand sperm DNA damage: Different reproductive effects on male fertility. Genes. 2019;**10**:105. DOI: 10.3390/genes10020105

[73] Ni W, Xiao S, Qiu X. Effect of sperm DNA fragmentation on clinical outcome of frozen-thawed embryo transfer and on blastocyst formation. PLoS One. 2014;**9**:e94956. DOI: 10.1371/journal.pone.0094956

[74] Dai X, Wang Y, Cao F. Sperm enrichment from poor semen samples by double density gradient centrifugation in combination with swim-up for IVF cycles. Scientific Reports. 2020;**10**:2286. DOI: 10.1038/s41598-020-59347-y

[75] Sun TC, Zhang Y, Li HT. Sperm DNA fragmentation index, as measured by sperm chromatin dispersion, might not predict assisted reproductive outcome. Taiwanese Journal of Obstetrics & Gynecology. 2018;**57**:493-498. DOI: 10.1016/j.tjog.2018.06.003

[76] Simon L, Zini A, Dyachenko A. A systematic review and meta-analysis to determine the effect of sperm DNA damage on in vitro fertilization and intracytoplasmic sperm injection outcome. Asian Journal of Andrology. 2017;**19**:80-90. DOI: 10.4103/1008-682X.182822

[77] Maheshwari A, McLernon D, Bhattacharya S. Cumulative live birth rate: Time for a consensus? Human Reproduction. 2015;**30**:2703-2707. DOI: 10.1093/humrep/dev263

[78] Malić VS, Stenqvist A, Bungum M. Sperm DNA fragmentation index and cumulative live birth rate in a cohort of 2,713 couples undergoing assisted reproduction treatment. Fertility and Sterility. 2021;**116**:1483-1490. DOI: 10.1016/j.fertnstert.2021.06.049

[79] Liang X, Duan R, Luo Q. Number of available embryos: A prediction tool for analyzing the effect of sperm DNA fragmentation on pregnancy outcome of patients undergoing IVF cycles from embryology. Andrologia. 2023;**2023**:1921515. DOI: 10.1155/2023/1921515

[80] Agarwal A, Majzoub A, Esteves SC. Clinical utility of sperm DNA fragmentation testing: Practice recommendations based on clinical scenarios. Translational Andrology and Urology. 2016;**5**:935-950. DOI: 10.21037/tau.2016.10.03

[81] Zini A. Are sperm chromatin and DNA defects relevant in the clinic? Systems Biology in Reproductive Medicine. 2011;**57**:78-85. DOI: 10.3109/19396368.2010.515704

[82] Esteves SC, Gosálvez J, López-Fernández C. Diagnostic accuracy of sperm DNA degradation index (DDSi)

as a potential noninvasive biomarker to identify men with varicocele-associated infertility. International Urology and Nephrology. 2015;**47**:1471-1477. DOI: 10.1007/s11255-015-1053-6

[83] Zhang F, Li J, Liang Z. Sperm DNA fragmentation and male fertility: A retrospective study of 5114 men attending a reproductive center. Journal of Assisted Reproduction and Genetics. 2021;**38**:1133-1141. DOI: 10.1007/s10815-021-02120-5

[84] Agarwal A, Farkouh A, Parekh N. Sperm DNA fragmentation: A critical assessment of clinical practice guidelines. World Journal of Mens Health. 2022;**40**:30-37. DOI: 10.5534/wjmh.210056

[85] Yoshiakwa-Terada K, Takeuchi H, Tachibana R. Age, sexual abstinence duration, sperm morphology, and motility are predictors of sperm DNA fragmentation. Reproductive Medicine and Biology. 2024;**23**:e12585. DOI: 10.1002/rmb2.12585

Chapter 6

# Phytochemicals of Natural Fruit Extract Rehabilitate Male Reproductive Health

*Syeda Nadia Ahmad and Khawaja Raees Ahmad*


## Abstract

Male infertility has become a global health issue nowadays. Insecticides damage the male reproductive system but can be rescued via the use of medicinal fruit extracts (MFEs). A number of experimental studies have shown that MFEs ameliorate testicular histopathologies induced by environmental (toxin) exposure in albino mice. MFEs show good capacity for testicular rehabilitation because of the presence of phytochemicals, especially phytosterols and natural antioxidants. Additionally, we have recently reported better survival rates and fertilizability of cryopreserved spermatozoa on the fortification of semen extenders with MFEs. On the basis of these findings, it is concluded that chemicals and insecticides are potential disruptors of spermatogenic activity and testicular microarchitecture *in vivo,* whereas the MFEs have shown excellent rehabilitative potentials in these contexts. Moreover, MFEs have also been shown to contribute to the post -hawed semen quality parameters.


**Keywords:** insecticides, MFEs, fertility, phytochemicals, natural antioxidants, medicinal fruits, interstitial tissue, seminiferous tubules

## 1. Introduction

Male reproductive system toxicity is becoming a hot issue of a current era because of the exposure to multiple environmental chemicals, insecticides, and toxins that lead to male infertility. Injury to the testicles, testicular cancer, hypogonadism, premature ejaculation, and azoospermia may also lead toward male infertility. Male infertility if addressed by xenobiotics, then it brings disturbances in the hormonal regulations, increases oxidative stress, causes cellular apoptosis in the testes [1]. Nowadays, insecticides used in the domestic and agricultural sectors have increased too much because they are considered to be safer than other pesticides [2]. Exposure to noxious chemicals brings degenerations in the testes lead to azoospermia, Sertoli cells necrosis, and damage in the spermatic cells and interstitial tissue. This stress triggers the rehabilitative activities in the male reproductive system and leads to rapid rehabilitation in the interstitial and spermatogenic tissue.



IntechOpen

### 1.1 Chemical and testicular damage

Carbon tetrachloride ($CCl_4$) is used in the production of refrigerants, foam-blowing agents, paints, plastics, and fumigants. It damages reproductive organs like testis [3]. It produces trichloromethyl ($CCl_3$) and trichloroperoxyl free radicals ($CCl_3O_2$) that lead to lipid peroxidation (reference). These free radicals damage the membranes of testicular cells. Biological exposure to $CCl_4$ and occupational applications has led to various fertility issues like impaired spermatogenesis, hormonal changes, and degeneration of various differentiating spermatozoa [4]. $CCl_4$ mainly targets the polyunsaturated fatty acids in the sperm membrane and causes lipid peroxidation [5]. Spermatozoa are highly sensitive because they are most vulnerable to oxidative stress and lack natural antioxidant enzymes like superoxide dismutase and glutathione transferases. Moreover, spermatozoa contain many mitochondria important for the constant supply of adenosine triphosphate (ATP) and propulsive movements. So, any sudden metabolic change may lead to oxidative stress [6]. The testicular smear and histological sections of the $CCl_4$ exposure showed obliterations of the interstitial cells, disturbances in spermatogenic cells, dislocations of developing spermatozoa, the presence of tailless sperms, larger-headed spermatids, and damage to the seminiferous tubules [7].

### 1.2 Pyrethroid insecticides and testicular damage

In general, pesticides like insecticides, herbicides, molluscicides, rodenticides, fungicides and nematicides, organochlorines, organophosphates, and carbamates act as endocrine disruptors which are responsible for the impairment of the male reproductive system and damage its physiology [8]. Insecticides like pyrethroids have two groups. Type I pyrethroids without alpha cyano moiety like permethrin, bifenthrin, allethrin, phenothrin, resmethrin, tefluthrin, tetramethrin, and fenvalerate and type II pyrethroids with alpha cyano moiety like cypermethrin, cyfluthrin, cyhalothrin, fenvalerate, fenpropathrin, flucythrinate, flumethrin, fluvalinate, tralomethrin, lambda-cyhalothrin, and deltamethrin. Mostly type II pyrethroids have been used due to their better efficiency and pest control. Unfortunately, these insecticides considered as most toxic to non-targeted organisms and result in severe damage to physiological processes and reproductive function when passed through the food chain [2]. The type II pyrethroids such as cypermethrin (CP), lambda-cyhalothrin (LN), deltamethrin, and permethrin have been extensively used in pest management all over the world [9]. These are mainly used to control mosquitos, spiders, mites, etc., and particularly the insect pests in major cereal crops and the fruits and vegetable fields. Unfortunately, their excessive dependency and use have been seen to bring infertility problems in males [7, 10]. Exposure to pyrethroid may bring damage to testicular interstitial tissue. Like exposure to CP shrinks the seminiferous tubules and produces wide interstitial. Another fluoridated pyrethroid insecticide LN causes the enlargement of seminiferous tubules via the retention of extracellular fluid in the interstitial spaces. The spermatogenic cells are also damaged by the exposure to both insecticides, but the mechanism of CP and LN toxicity is different in both insecticides. Exposure to CP causes shrinkage of seminiferous tubules that shows fluid retention only in the interstitial tissue with deformed tubules in terms of wavy tubular margins. However, exposure to LN insecticide brings retention of extracellular fluid inside seminiferous tubules. Pyrethroids directly damage the male reproductive organs, that is, testes and accessory organs, that is, epididymis and vas deferens.

They also affect morphology of testes, epididymis, and vas deferens. Further research must be conducted in the future to explore sperm abnormalities and male infertility problems caused by direct exposure to fluorinated and non-fluorinated pyrethroid insecticides. Future prospects may also include the therapeutic effects of extra virgin olive oil on interstitial tissue, seminiferous tubules, epididymis, and vas deferens [1].

### 1.3 Heavy metal and testicular damage

Heavy metals cause health problems and lead (Pb) poisoning is one of these global issues. Lead exposure brings alterations in spermatogenesis, and sperm functional parameters and causes serious fluctuations in circulating reproductive hormones. Pb causes cellular vacuolations, disturbs mitosis, alters cellular proliferation of Sertoli cells, and brings apoptosis in the seminiferous tubules. Pb in high concentration interrupts spermatozoa, and reduce the number of spermatogonia and Leydig cells [11]. Similarly, cadmium (Cd) is a toxic heavy metal that affects the male reproductive system. Cadmium accumulation in reproductive organs leads to decreased testicular weight and induces cellular necrosis in the testis that leads to a significant reduction in the number of germ and Sertoli cells along with a generally decreased production of androgens and gonadotropins [12]. Chromium (Cr) is the most common effluent of textiles, used in the paints industry, chrome plating, stainless steel welding, and leather tannery industries. Cd exposure disturbs the normal process of spermatogenesis and its anatomy. Cd induces lipid peroxidation and reduces the functioning of enzymatic. Cr deteriorates sperm formation; shrinks the diameter of seminiferous tubules, and decrease sperm motility and a number of germ cells. Moreover, Cr exposure also decreases the number of epididymal spermatozoa together with increased abnormality of sperm. Cr causes loss of interstitial tissue, spermatogonia and spermatocytes [13].

### 1.4 Insect pest, MFEs, and male fertility

Antioxidants are chelating agents that scavenge free oxygen radicals (reactive oxygen species [ROS]) and save cell membranes, endomembrane system, DNA, and various enzyme co-enzymes systems and metal ions form ROS attack. $CCl_4$ damaged the interstitial tissue and spermatogenic cells, causing cellular obliterations and leaving wide empty spaces between the Leydig cells. It brings lipid peroxidation in the cellular membranes and leads to cellular necrosis of Sertoli cells [7]. The recent trends of research indicate the ameliorative potentials of medicinal fruit extracts (MFEs) like *Basella alba*, *Solanum nigrum*, *Ficus carica,* and *Grewia asiatica* against the toxic implications of noxious chemical agents like $CCl_4$ as indicated in the experimental exposure-related organ pathologies (**Figures 1** and **2**; **Table 1** and 2) [10]. It is worth mentioning here that FE of Jambul (*Syzygium cumini*) has been seen to significantly improve various quality parameters of the cryopreserved bovine semen, through the maintenance of sperm membrane integrity, motility, and fertilizability [11]. MFEs of *S. cumini* has a unique blend of flavonoids, polyphenols, and variety of anthocyanins that act as an exceptional antioxidant. These antioxidants have multiple hydroxyl groups, conjugated double bonds, and electron-releasing capacity, reducing and non-reducing sugars that protect the developing spermatozoa from oxidative stress. These MFEs may serve as an excellent cryoprotective agent against cryogenic injuries. Phytosterols of these MFE like beta-sitosterol gave protection to

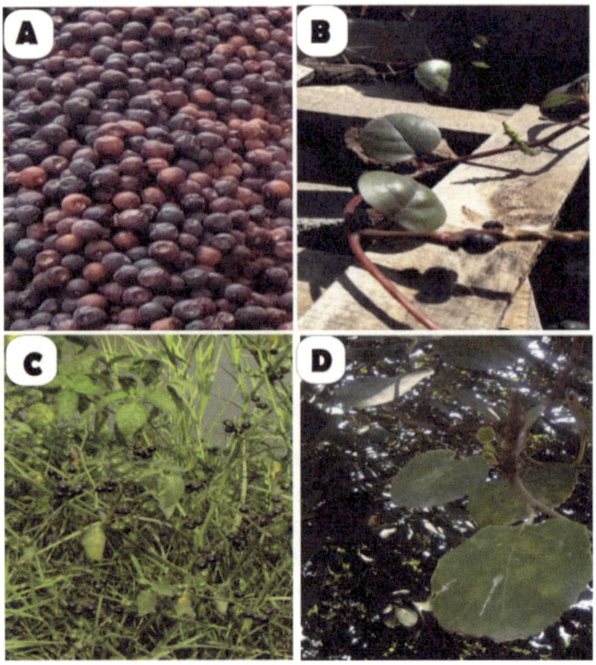

**Figure 1.**
*Fruits have active phytochemicals, (A):* Grewia asiatica*; (B):* Basella alba*; (C):* Solanum nigrum*; and (D):* Ficus carica.

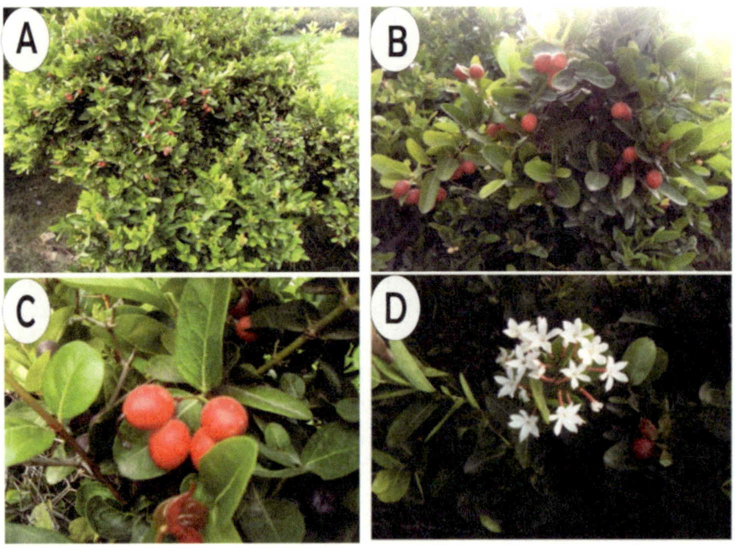

**Figure 2.**
Carissa carandus *plant. (A):* Carissa carandus *is ever green shrub consist of root, stem, flower and red to dark purple fruit; (B):* Carissa carandus *fruits; (C): Ripe Karanda fruit; and (D):* Carissa carandus *flowers.*

the sperm plasma membrane and enhance its integrity. MFEs of *S. cumini* enhance sperm membrane integrity and fertilizability leads to an increase in a mean number of progressively motile sperms and whirling spermatozoa. Fruits of *S. cumini* plant

| Fruits | Phytochemicals | Particular antioxidants of fruits |
|---|---|---|
| Malabar spinach<br>*Basella alba* | Minerals; Anthocyanins: Betacyanins; Flavonoids: Kaempferol; Acids; Phenolic acids; Sterols: Beta-sitosterol, Saponins, Glycosides, Coumarin, Anthracene, Glycoside, ß-carotene, Luteolin, Zeaxanthin. | Betacyanin, Beta-sitosterol, Kaempferol |
| Phalsa<br>*Grewia asiatica* | Vitamins; Fatty acids; Minerals: Sodium, Cobalt, Zinc, Manganese; Anthocyanins: Cyanidin, pelargonidin; Oils; Amino acids; Phenolic acids; Steroids: Kaempferol, β-sitosterol, Stigmasterol, Campesterol; Tocopherols. | Anthocyanidins, β-sitosterol, Stigmasterol, Naringenin |
| *Mako*<br>*Solanum nigrum* | Vitamins; Minerals; Organic acids; Lipids; Anthocyanins; Glycosides; Glycoalkaloids: Solanine; Alkaloids: Indole terpenoid and purine; Polyphenols: Gallic acid, Rutin; Steroidal saponin, Sterols alkaloids, Solamargine, Solasonine, α and β- solanigrine; Non-saponins. | Alkaloids, Tannins, Gallic acid, Solanine and sterols, caffeic acid |
| Fig latex<br>*Ficus carica* | Vitamins; Terpenoid; Anthocyanins; Phenols; Acids; Phenolic acids: Ferulic acid; Polyphenols; Sterols: β-sitosterol, campesterol, Psoralen. | β-sitosterol, Campesterol, Stigmasterol, Fucosterol, Pelargonidin |

**Table 1.**
*Most important phytochemical ingredients of MFE's of* Basella alba, Grewia asiatica, Solanum nigrum, *and* Ficus carica *[10, 14].*

are adapted to survive at high temperatures, in arid, sandy, and rocky areas. Due to their survival under harsh environmental conditions, MFE possesses huge amounts of antioxidants, for example, anthocyanins, flavonoids, polyphenols, and phytosterols such as b-sitosterol and stigmasterol [6]. MFEs of *S. cumini* and *Morus alba* promote the process of spermatogenesis against Pb-exposed mice testes. Both MFEs partially rehabilitate the interstitial tissue and enhances the number of spermatogonia [11]. Fruit extract of *Basella rubra* enhance frozen thawed ram sperm's motility, velocity, and membrane integrity [15]. MFEs of *B. rubra* biologically support sperm metabolism and survival and hence are considered to be crucial components against cryoinjuries during the process of sperm cryopreservation. Its MFEs contain active carbohydrates, amino acids, ellagic acid, flavonoids, unsaturated fatty acids, vitamins, anthocyanins, quercetin, folate, and carotenoids that support the sperms and enhance its stability [16].

*Morus nigra* fruit extract has been found to significantly improve sperm survival rate, progressive motility, and *in vitro* fertilizability [16]. MFEs of *Morus nigra* has enormous amounts of phenolics, flavanoids, anthocyanins, cardiac glycosides, amino acids, saponins, tannins, and sugars that have antioxidant potential. These phytochemicals show excellent cryoprotective abilities and improve sperm motility [15]. In the same context, the extra virgin olive oil (EVO) has been found to effectively ameliorate the male reproductive anomalies and enhance male fertility [17]. EVO has an immune-protective capacity and thus can be used against insecticide-inflicted testicular histopathologies [1].

In the same way, the testicular anomalies caused by the exposure of Pb can be recovered by the use of Jambul (*Syzygium cumini*) and White mulberry (*Morus alba*) fruit extracts [18]. Natural plant fruit extract (NPFEs) of similar fruit extract of *Basella rubra* has been found to rehabilitate the compromises of the male reproductive system on account of pesticide exposures [2]. Similarly, MFEs of *S. cumini* show rehabilitative potential in the testes against Cd-induced exposure [19].

| Histological findings | | | Groups | | | |
|---|---|---|---|---|---|---|
| | | | **Effect of MFE's of** *Basella alba* | **Effect of MFE's of** *Solanum nigrum* | **Effect of MFE's of** *Ficus carica* | **Effect of MFE's of** *Grewia asiatica* |
| Histopathological effects | Seminiferous tubule | Shrinkage in seminiferous tubules | -- | ++++ | -- | -- |
| | | Disrupted arrangement of the spermatogenic cells | -- | ++++ | + | -- |
| | Interstitial tissue | Leydig cells necrosis | -- | -- | -- | -- |
| | | Focal degenerations in the interstitial tissue | + | -- | -- | -- |
| Rehabilitative potential | Seminiferous tubule | Rehabilitation of the spermatogenic cell arrangement (whirl) in the seminiferous tubules | *** | * | *** | *** |
| | Interstitial tissue | Interstitial tissue regeneration and rehabilitation | *** | *** | *** | *** |
| Regenerative potential | Spermatogenesis | Spermatogenic cells regeneration | *** | × | *** | *** |
| | | Luminal population of spermatozoa | * | × | ** | *** |
| | Interstitial tissue | Interstitial tissue regeneration | *** | *** | *** | *** |

++++: *Most prominent effect,* +: *Less moderate effect,*--: *Little or no effect,* ***: *Excellent rehabilitative/Regenerative response,* **: *Very good rehabilitative/Regenerative response,**: *Fairly good rehabilitative/Regenerative response,* ×: *Little or no rehabilitative/Regenerative response.*

**Table 2.**
*The curative and regenerative potential of Basella alba, Solanum nigrum, Ficus carica and Grewia asiatica MFEs.*

## 2. Role of phytochemical to boost male fertility

Herbal products or naturopathic treatments are preferably used for medicinal purposes due to cost effectiveness, easy intake, high success rate, and less or no side effects. Moreover, society cannot afford the heavy surgical, low success rate, risky procedures, greater side effects, and treatment costs. Hence, societies are shifting from synthetic medications to herbal formulations [20].

MFEs rehabilitate the testes and speed up the process of steroidogenesis and spermatogenesis, realign sperm-producing cells of seminiferous tubules, re-arrange the whirls of spermatogonia near the basement membrane. MFEs of *Basella alba*, *Ficus carica* and *Grewia asiatica* have unique blends of phytosterols, for example, sitosterol, stigmasterol, and campesterol (**Table 1**). These phytosterols mimic the function of male sex hormones and promote anabolic activities in the male reproductive system. Mechanism of testicular rehabilitation involves the active role of pericytes near the margins of the seminiferous tubules. These pericytes became active by the exposure of MFE's androgenic phytosterols and proliferate during testicular rehabilitation. MFEs of *Ficus carica* show fastest pace of testicular rehabilitation of the interstitial tissue, increase androgen secretion level, and eventually lead to enhancement of the processes of meiosis and spermiogenesis [7]. Fruit extract of *Basella alba* contains certain phytosterols like kaempferol and beta-sitosterol that are capable of reducing stress-related immuno-cellular responses (**Table 1**) [14]. Additionally, *Besila rubera* fruit extract (BR-FE) contains cyanine, gomphrenin I and III, minerals, folic acid, ascorbic acid, phenols, polyphenols, flavonoids, anthocyanins, all of which have distinct pharmacological benefits [21]. In BR-FE polyphenols, ellagic acid, flavonoids, anthocyanins, quercetin, and kaempferol, may play a role as powerful antioxidants during semen freeze–thaw processes (**Table 3**) [22].

Mulberry fruit extract contains phytochemicals like phenol, flavonoid, anthocyanin (cyanidin 3-O-glucoside, cyanidin 3-O-rutinoside, pelargonidin 3-O-glucoside, pelargonidin 3-O-rutinoside), benzoic acid derivatives (protocatechuic acid, p-hydroxybenzoic acid, vanillic acid), cinnamic acid derivatives (Caffeic acid, ferulic acid, chlorogenic acid), and ascorbic acid have ROS protective capacities [23].

Similarly, the MFEs of *Grewia asiatica* and *Ficus carica* contain phytosterols, for example, campesterol and stigmasterol [24] and the EVO contains precious phenolic compounds, oleocanthal, oleuropein, hydroxytyrosol, and tyrosol that enhance male fertility [15]. The *Syzygium cumini* fruit extract has been found to have bioactive phytochemicals like anthocyanins, tannins, raffinose, petunidin, and the gallic, malic and citric acids that improve testicular architectural mutilations [25].

The active photo-medicinal ingredient of *Morus alba*-Fruit extract (MA-FE) that protect reproductive cells is amino acids, fatty acids, vitamins, minerals, quercetin, and chlorogenic acid [26]. The MFE of *Basella rubra* has healthy effects on male reproductive function. It is reported to enhance serum level of testosterone and concentration of spermatozoa in the lumen of the seminiferous tubules due to the presence of bioactive pyhtochemicals like β-cyanin, gomphrenin I, gomphrenin II and III [27]. NPFEs *Carissa carandus* (Karonda) contain natural phytochemicals like carisol, epimer of α-amyrin, carissic acid, linalool, β-caryophyllene, ascorbic acid, carissone, carindone, and β-sitosterol that show anti-inflammatory and andro-protective activities that produce reproductive health effects in the experimental animals (mice) [28].

| Phytochemicals of *Basella rubra* MFE's | Function |
|---|---|
| Sinapic acid | Perform better scavenging agent |
| Ferulic acid | Work as antioxidant |
| Coumaric acid | Antioxidant and anti-inflammatory |
| Chlorogenic acid | Antioxidant activities |
| Myricetin | Antioxidant and anti-inflammatory |
| Quercetin | Antioxidant and anti-inflammatory |
| Luteolin | Antioxidant |
| Kaempferol | Antioxidant |
| Vitamin A | Essential for spermatogenesis |
| Vitamin C | Protect spermatogenesis |

**Table 3.**
*Phytochemicals of* Basella rubra *fruit and their functions [22].*

MFEs of *Morus nigra* or black mulberry serve as excellent antioxidants because of the high concentration of anthocyanins than of all the mulberries [13]. MFE of *Fragaria vesca* has high antioxidant activity due to the presence of bioactive ingredients like ellagitannins, flavonoids, calcium, potassium, magnesium, iron, phosphorous, pro-anthocyanidins, ascorbic acid, sucrose, fructose, glucose, and phenolic acids polyphenols. In comparison with garden strawberries (*Fragaria ananassa*), *Fragaria vesca* MFEs have higher vitamin C, total ellagic acids, and total phenolic levels. The active MFEs of *Fragaria vesca* in the extender chelate the harmful nascent oxygen produced in the sperm. At thawing, ROS of sperms protected by the polyphenols, for example, anthocyanins and ellagic acids of *Fragaria vesca* mainly [29].

## 3. Testicular rehabilitation by MFEs

Histological picture of testes shows round seminiferous tubules covered by a basement membrane. Seminiferous tubules have spermatogenic cells like spermatogonia, spermatocytes, spermatids and spermatozoa in central whirls. Healthy and normal interstitial tissue surrounds each seminiferous tubule (**Figure 3**). Seminiferous tubules after $CCl_4$ exposure show a deformed shape. As well as the internal arrangement of spermatogenic cells and spermatozoa was found scattered and poorly differentiated (**Figure 4**). Excellent regenerative events were observed after exposure to MFEs of *Grewia asiatica*. Here lumen of seminiferous tubules was occupied with an enormous number of maturing spermatozoa. Regeneration of interstitial tissue was also observed from the pericytes resulting in the reappearance of Leydig cells. Regenerative events were quite obvious after exposure to *Ficus carica* MFE's. The arrangement of spermatogenic cells was appropriate with healthier interstitial tissue. Partial rehabilitative ultrastructural architectural arrangements were observed after exposure of MFEs of *Basella alba*. The healthy interstitial tissue was observed with many regenerating Leydig cells. Surprisingly, after exposure to MFE's *Solanum nigrum* size of the seminiferous tubules was reduced with variable polygonal irregular margins. The spermatogenic cells and spermatid proper alignment were disturbed.

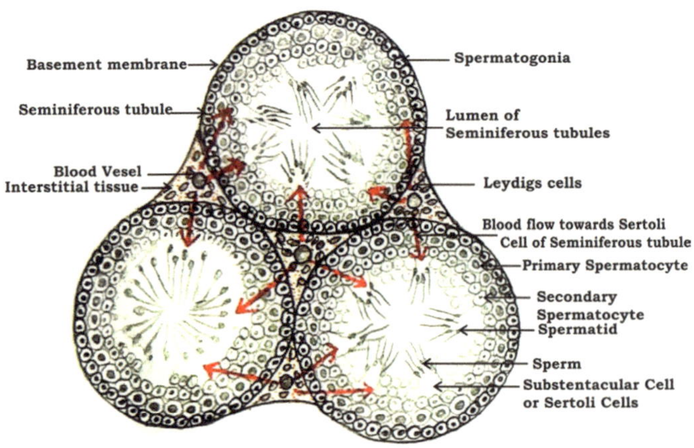


**Figure 3.**
*Anatomical regions of mouse testes consisting of seminiferous tubules.*

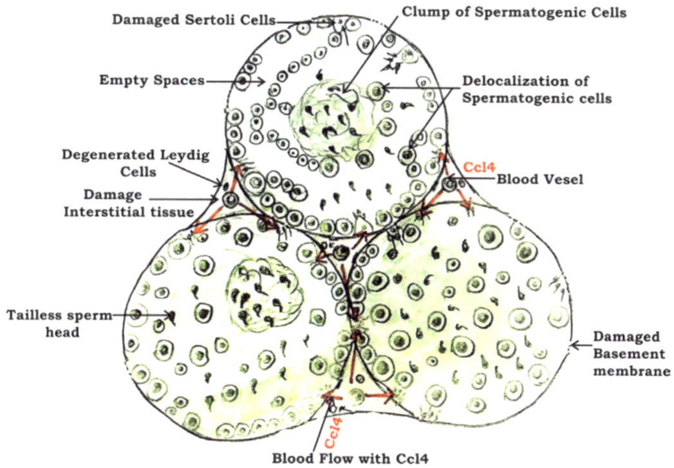


**Figure 4.**
*Pathological signs observed in $CCl_4$ exposure group of mouse testes.*

All seminiferous tubules were devoid of differentiating spermatozoa and necrotic interstitial tissue. However, the marginal cells or pericytes of the interstitial tissue were undisturbed (**Figures 5** and **6**; **Table 2**) [7].

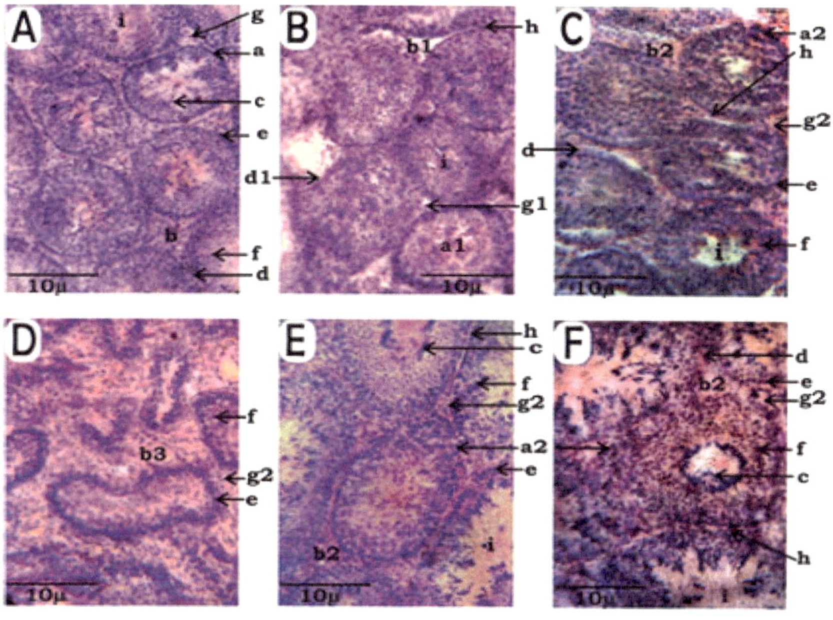


**Figure 5.**
*Histological sections of testes (400X, H and E-stained sections). (A): Control (Reference), (B): CCl4, C: CCl4 + MFE of* Basella alba*, (D): CCl4+ MFE of* Solnum nigrum*, (E): CCl4 + MFE of* Grewia asiatica*, and (F): CCl4 + MFE of* Ficus carica*, a: Normal seminiferous tubules, a1: Damaged seminiferous tubules, a2: Regenerated seminiferous tubules, b: Normal interstitial tissue, b1: Degenerated interstitial tissue, b2: Regenerated interstitial tissue, b3: Fibrosis of interstitial tissue, c: Normal sperm distribution pattern, d: Basement membrane, d1: Damaged basement membrane, e: Spermatogonia, f: Spermatocytes, g: Leydig cells, g1: Degenerated Leydig cells, g2: Regenerated Leydig cells, h: Pericytes, and i: Lumen in seminiferous tubules.*

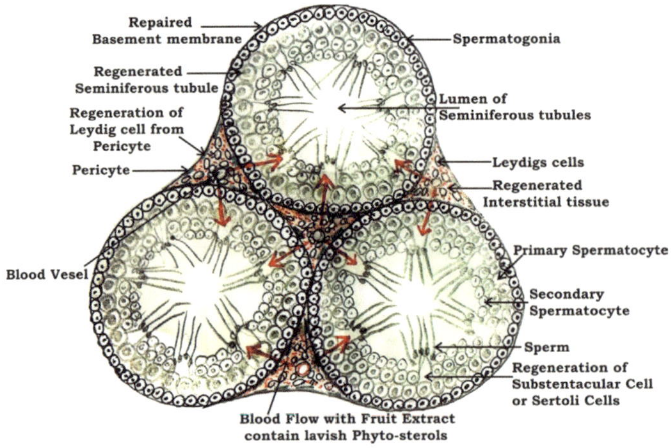


**Figure 6.**
*Shows testicular recovery and rehabilitative seminiferous tubules by means of fruit extract.*

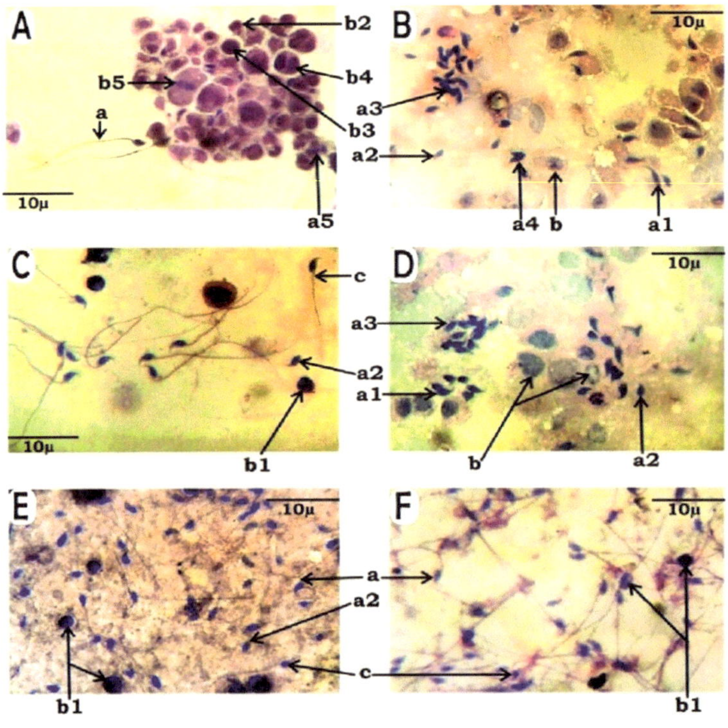


**Figure 7.**
*Testicular smears (400X magnification, Hematoxylin and eosin-stained sections). (A): Control (Reference), (B): CCl4, (C): CCl4 + MFE of* Basella alba, *(D): CCl4+ MFE of* Solanum nigrum, *(E): CCl4 +* Grewia asiatica, *and (F): CCl4 +* Ficus carica, *a: Normal sperms with parakeet beak-shaped head, small neck, middle piece, and well developed straight and long tail, a1: Tailless sperm spermatids with crow beak-shaped head, a2: Micronuclei spermatid head, a3: Cluster of spermatids with probably halted spermiogenesis, a4: Two headed spermatid, a5: Normal spermatids, b: Necrotizing spermatogenic cells (Spermatogonia andspermatocytes), b1: Healthy spermatogeniccells (Spermatogonia andspermatocytes), b2:Normalspermatogonia,b3:Primary spermatocyte, b4: Secondary spermatocyte, b5: Mitotic spindle of primary spermatocyte, and c: Still sperms with normal tail.*

## 4. Spermatozoa rehabilitation by MFEs

Testicular smears show a large number of spermatozoa with parakeet beak-shaped heads, a curved and elongated acrosome, and a middle piece with a long straight tail (**Figure 3**). After $CCl_4$ exposure less mature spermatozoa were observed with rare clumps of interstitial cells (**Figure 4**). After exposure to MFEs of *Basella alba* many maturing and mature spermatozoa and some aggregations of interstitial cells were seen. Surprisingly, after exposure to MFE's *Solanum nigrum* the situation seems to be still worse in terms of a large number of necrotizing spermatids with no matured and maturing spermatozoa that indicate almost complete loss of spermatogenesis. Maximum spermatids were observed after exposure to MFEs of *Grewia asiatica.* Almost the same results were observed after exposure to MFEs of *Basella alba.* Exposure of *Ficus carica* to MFEs reveals the presence of healthy spermatogenic cells, maturing spermatids, matured spermatozoa, and a few clumps of interstitial cells (**Figures 6** and 7) [7].

The signs of recovery from testicular histopathologies were observed in *Grewia asiatica*, *Basella alba,* and *Ficus carica* against $CCl_4$ exposure that include regeneration in the interstitial tissue and realignment of spermatogenic cells. The *Grewia asiatica*, *Basella alba,* and *Ficus carica* contain a variety of phytosterols like androstenediol, androstenedione, dehydroepiandrosterone, dihydrotestosterone, and testosterone. All phytosterol mimics the role of male sex hormones and promote the cellular anabolic activities in the testes that lead to hypertrophy in the spermatogenic and interstitial cells of Leydig's and ultimately contribute toward the rehabilitation of spermatogenesis and the male hormone production (**Figure 6**).

## 5. Micrometric effects of the used MFEs

The micrometric data of testicular sections also indicate significant ($p < 0.05$) decline in the mean number of spermatogonia along the length (1 μ) of the basement membrane in $CCl_4$ (1.14 ± 0.14) than rest of the four MFE's *Solanum nigrum*, *Ficus carica*, *Grewia asiatica,* and *Basella alba* (1.79 ± 0.16, 1.71 ± 0.15, 1.53 ± 0.16, 1.30 ± 0.12, 1.29 ± 0.11, respectively). Interestingly the mean cross-sectional area (CSA) of seminiferous tubules remained significantly ($p < 0.05$) higher in $CCl_4$ than *Grewia asiatica* and *Solanum nigrum* MFE and the use of *Ficus carica* MFE showed significant CSA. Whereas the CSA of sperm head remained significantly ($p < 0.05$) higher after exposure to MFE of *Solanum nigrum* (12.13 ± 1.06 $\mu m^2$) than the other three MFEs that are *Ficus carica*, *Basella alba,* and *Grewia asiatica* (6.99 ± 0.27, 6.66 ± 0.41, 6.06 ± 0.19 $\mu m^{2,}$ respectively). Contrarily, the mean tail length of sperm remained significantly ($p < 0.05$) lower in the *Solanum nigrum* MFE group (5.04 ± 0.86 μm) than rest of all MFE's *Grewia asiatica*, *Ficus carica,* and *Basella alba* (32.82 ± 1.64, 48.99 ± 0.93, 56.67 ± 0.89 μm, respectively). Likewise, the mean number of the seminiferous tubules/unit area (35,840 $\mu m^2$) remained significantly ($p < 0.05$) lower in *Ficus carica* MFE exposed group (2.18 ± 0.05) than the rest of all MFE's *Grewia asiatica* (3.42 ± 0.07), *Solanum nigrum* (5.91 ± 0.07), and *Basella alba* (3.41 ± 0.06) [7].

## 6. Mechanism of testicular rehabilitation by MFEs

Activation of the dormant marginal pericytes of the seminiferous tubules rehabilitates the functional Leydig's cells. Pericytes show proliferation and

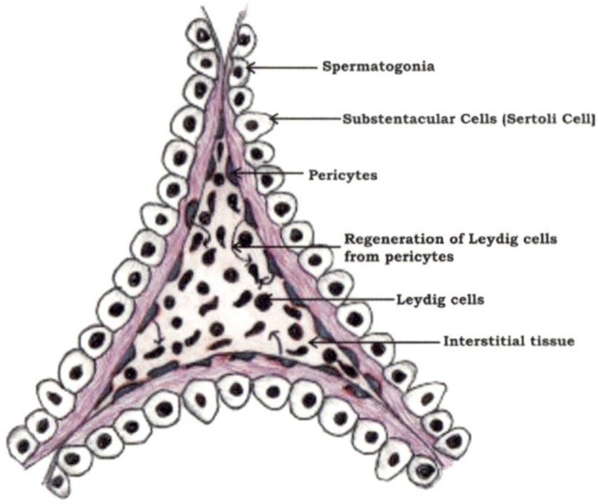


**Figure 8.**
*Interstitial tissue rehabilitation by progenitor cells "pericytes".*

maturational activities that help in the restoration of interstitial tissue via mitotic activities triggered by phytosterols (**Figures 8** and **9**) [30]. MFE's of *Solanum nigrum* show extreme shrinkage of the seminiferous tubules due to the presence of anti-steroidogenic ingredient solasonine which damage the surviving spermatogonia and



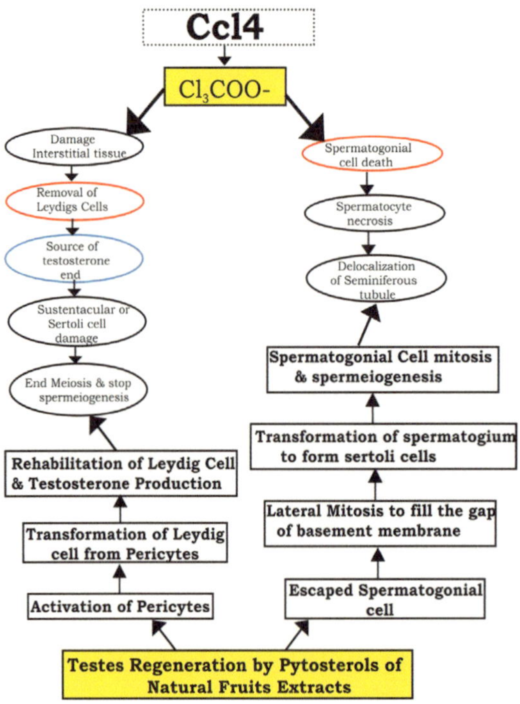


**Figure 9.**
*Flow chart shows that oxidative stress created by any toxicant, e.g., $CCl_4$ and MFEs as antioxidants involved during testes rehabilitation.*

halts the process of spermatogenesis. Solasonine is lavishly present in the MFE of *Solanum nigrum* which damages the process of steroidogenesis and interfere with the rehabilitation of the interstitial tissue [31]. Partial rehabilitation in spermatogenic cells by MFE's of *Grewia asiatica* and *Basella alba* were mainly attributable to their precious phytosterols (**Table 1**). Best rehabilitatory activities of the spermatogenic cells was seen by the use of MFE's of *Grewia asiatica* which should be attributed to its phytosterols present in MFE, which helped to enhance spermatogenesis. A similar blend of phytosterols was present in *Basella alba* MFE (**Table 1**) that enhanced the number of mature spermatozoa in the testicular smear. It is because of the presence of a variety of antioxidants in the *Basella alba* MFE that leads to the rapid rehabilitation of interstitial tissue (**Figure 7**; **Table 1**). MFE of *Ficus carica* latex also contains a variety of the precious antioxidants that enhance the number of mature spermatozoa (**Figure 7**; **Table 1**). All MFEs help in the rapid rehabilitation of the interstitial tissue that increases natural androgen secretions, ultimately leading to complete rehabilitation of testicular mitosis, meiosis, and spermatogenesis (**Figure 9**). *Basella alba*, *Grewia asiatica*, *Solanum nigrum,* and *Ficus carica* MFE's contain precious ingredients like amino acids, sugars, vitamins, polyphenols, anthocyanins, and phytosterols (**Table 1**). These MFPs boost up the natural pace of the rehabilitative activities of the testis (**Table 2**).

## 7. Conclusion

The aforementioned literature indicates that the environmental chemicals, insecticides, pesticides, and heavy metals are potential disruptors of spermatogenesis and sperm viability in testes. However, as these adverse conditions were partially reversed by the post-treatment of various natural plant fruit extracts, it indicates the rehabilitative and rescuing potential of these fruits. It is thus suggested that the MFEs can be used as potential remedial dietary substances against the environmental toxins. Furthermore, it is suggested that more research on MFEs should be on clinical trials to replace these MFEs with synthetic products to enhance fertility rates. So that the quality of life should be improved.

## Acknowledgements

Authors are thankful to the authorities of the University of Sargodha and University of Chakwal for the logistic and research facilities to conduct animal trials as indicated in many of the abovementioned references. We are also thankful to the authors and their institutions (other than the University of Chakwal and University of Sargodha) whose research work is mentioned as a reference in this chapter.

The authorship criteria are listed in our Authorship Policy. Available from: https://www.intechopen.com/page/authorship-policy.

This section of your manuscript may also include funding information.

## Conflict of interest

The authors declare that they have no conflict of interest.

## Appendices and nomenclature

| | |
|---|---|
| MFE's | Medicinal fruit extracts |
| BR-FE | *Basella rubra* fruit extract |
| EVO | Extra virgin olive oil |
| MA-FE | *Morus alba* fruit extract |
| CP | Cypermethrin |
| LN | Lambda-cyhalothrin |
| Pb | Lead |
| Cr | Chromium |

## Author details

Syeda Nadia Ahmad[1*] and Khawaja Raees Ahmad[2]

1 Department of Zoology, University of Chakwal, Chakwal, Pakistan

2 Department of Zoology, University of Sargodha, Sargodha, Pakistan

*Address all correspondence to: nadia.ahmad@uoc.edu.pk

## References

[1] Kanwal N, Ahmad KR, Ahmad SN, Suleman S, Ahmed SA, Kanwal MA, et al. Andrological pathologies of fluoridated and non-fluoridated pyrethroid insecticide exposure in mice. Fluoride. 2023;**56**(4):512-529

[2] Ahmad SN, Sattar HA, Kanwal MA, Inayat I, Suleman S, Younis A, et al. Protective effects of Basella rubra against fluoridated pyrethroid insecticide induced reproductive health toxicity in mice. Fluoride. 2023;**56**(e251):1-8

[3] Sherry D, McCulloch A, Liang Q, Reimann S, Newman PA. Current sources of carbon tetrachloride (CCl4) in our atmosphere. Environmental Research Letters. 2018;**13**:24004

[4] Elsawy H, Badr GM, Sedky A, Abdallah BM, Alzahrani AM, Abdel-Moneim AM. Rutin ameliorates carbon tetrachloride (CCl4) induced hepatorenal toxicity and hypogonadism in male rats. PeerJ. 2019;**7**:e7011

[5] Foaud MA, Kamel AH, Abd El-Monem DD. The protective effect of N-acetyl cysteine against carbon tetrachloride toxicity in rats. Journal of Basic and Applied Zoology. 2018;**79**:14

[6] Sulman S, Kanwal MA, Malik F, Ali R, Siddique S, Kanwal N, et al. Jambul (Syzygium cumini) pulp extract enhances viability, motility, and in vitro fertilizability of cryopreserved bovine semen. Biopreservation and Biobanking. Feb 2021;**19**(1):53-59. DOI: 10.1089/bio.2020.0061. Epub 2020 Oct 20

[7] Ahmad SN, Ahmad KR, Abdullah U, Malik F, Ali R, Amir-ud-din U, et al. Basella alba, Grewia asiatica, Solanum nigrum and Ficus carica fruit extracts ameliorate the testicular histopathology induced by CCl4 exposure in albino mice: An experimental study. International Journal of Reproductive BioMedicine. 2022;**20**:101-110

[8] Ravula AR, Yenugu S. Long term oral administration of a mixture of pyrethroids affects reproductive function in rats. Reproductive Toxicology. 2019;**89**:1-12

[9] Guillem-Amat A, Lopez-Errasquin E, Castells-Sierra J, Sanchez L, Ortego F. Current situation and forecasting of resistance evolution to lambda-cyhalothrin in Spanish medfly populations. Pest Management Science. 2022;**78**(4):1341-1355

[10] Djouaka R, Soglo MF, Kusimo MO, Adéoti R, Talom A, Zeukeng F, et al. The rapid degradation of Lambda-Cyhalothrin makes treated vegetables relatively safe for consumption. International Journal of Environmental Research and Public Health. 2018;**15**(7):1536. DOI: 10.3390/ijerph15071536

[11] Santhosh KR, Asha DS. Lead toxicity on male reproductive system and its mechanism: A review. Research Journal of Pharmacy and Technology. 2018;**1**:1228-1232

[12] Shimada H, Narumi R, Nagano M, Yasurake A, Waalkes MP, Imamura Y. Strain difference of cadmium-induced testicular toxicity in inbred Wistar-Imamichi and fisher 344 rats. Archives of Toxicology. 2009;**83**:647-652

[13] Ahmad SN, Ahmad K, Jabeen K, Kanwal MA, Inayat I, Suleman S, et al. Amelioration by Morus Nigra fruit extract on testes, seminiferous tubules

and spermatic cells by chromium induced Histopathologies in mice. Journal of Bioresource Management. 2014;**11**(2):186-193

[14] Singh A, Dubey PK, Chaurasiya R, Mathur N, Kumar G, Bharati S. Indian spinach: An underutilized perennial leafy vegetable for nutritional security in developing world. Energy, Ecology and Environment. 2018;**3**:1007

[15] Ali M, Suleman S, Inayat I, Ahmad SN, Kanwal MA, Ahmad KR, et al. Fortification of extender with Basella rubra fruit extract enhances the cryosurvival of ram semen. Biopreservation and Biobanking. Feb 2024;**22**(1):46-50. DOI: 10.1089/bio.2022.0191. Epub 2023 May 8

[16] Suleman S, Kanwal MA, Ali R, Kanwal N, Yasmeen S, Mehmood MY, et al. Morus nigra fruit extract safeguards frozen thawed bovine sperm parameters. Iranian Journal of Applied Animal Sciences. 2023;**13**(2):267-275

[17] Ashry M, Galal EL, Sahra D, Abdel-Wahhab KG, Abdelsalam ME, Mourad HH, et al. Saussurea costus extract has anti-inflammatory, antioxidant, and hormonal effects against testicular toxicity induced by oxaliplatin in male albino rats. Iranian Journal of Toxicology. 2022;**16**(2):83-90

[18] Kanwal MA, Mehmood A, Anjum A, Inayat I, Ahmad SN, Suleman S, et al. Ameliorative effects of Syzygium cumini and Morus alba fruit extract on the testicular histopathology of lead exposed mice. Pakistan Journal of Scientific and Industrial Research, For Series B: Biolological Sciences. 2023;**66B**(3):249-254

[19] Inayat I, Ahmad SN, Batool H, Younis A, Abbas T, Batool S, et al. Mitigations of Syzygium cummini fruit extract on CdCl2 induced histopathological changes in laboratory mouse epididymids. Egyptian Academic Journal of Biological Sciences D. Histology and Histochemistry. 2019;**12**(1):48-58

[20] Chorosho SH, Malik N, Panesar G, Kumari P, Jangra S, Kaur R, et al. Phytochemicals: Alternative for infertility treatment and associated conditions. Oxidative Medicine and Cellular Longevity. 2023;**2023**:1327562

[21] Kumar PC, Oberoi HS, Azeez S. Basella-an underutilized green leafy vegetable with a potential for functional food development. Food Reviews International. 2022;**38**(Suppl. 1):456-473

[22] Singh M, Kumari R, Kotecha M. Basellarubralinn: A review. International Journal of Ayurveda and Pharmaceutical Chemistry. 2016;**5**(1):206-223

[23] Sanchez-Salcedo EM, Mena P, Garcia-Viguera C, Martínez JJ, Hernandez F. Phytochemical evaluation of white (Morusalba L.) and black (Morusnigra L.) mulberry fruits, a starting point for the assessment of their beneficial properties. Journal of Functional Foods. 2015;**12**:399-408

[24] Asghar W, Khalid N, Nazir W, Farooq M, Ahmed I. Phalsa (Grewia asiatica L) fruit berry a promising functional food ingredient: A comprehensive review. Journal of Berry Research. 2019;**9**:179-193

[25] Singh B, Singh JP, Kaur A, Singh N. Insights into the phenolic compounds present in jambolan (Syzygium cumini) along with their health promoting effects. International Journal of Food Science and Technology. 2018;**53**:2431-2447

[26] Yuan O, Zhao L. The mulberry (Morus alba) fruit-a review of characteristic components and health benefits. Journal of Agriculture of Food Chemistry. 2017;**65**:10383-10394

[27] Reddy GJ, Madhavi TR, Rao CA, Nithya SN. An updated phytochemical and pharmacological review on Malabar spinach (Basella alba or Basella rubra). GSC Biological and Pharmaceutical Sciences. 2023;**24**(2):161-169

[28] Dutta S. Assessment of acute anti-inflammatory effect of Carissa carandas leaf extracts in wistar albino rats. Journal of Advanced Pharmacy Education and Research. 2015;**5**:40-43

[29] Ahmad KR, Suleman S, Malik F, Kanwal MA, Ahmad SN, Yasmeen S, et al. Supplemental effect of wild strawberry (Fragaria vesca) pulp extract in extender to enhance quality attributes of cryopreserved bovine sperms. Reproduction and Breeding. 2024;**2024**(4):179-184

[30] Ye L, Li X, Li L, Chen H, Ge RS. Insights into the development of the adult Leydig cell lineage from stem Leydig cells. Frontiers in Physiology. 2017;**8**:430

[31] Wang Y, Xiang L, Yi X, He X. Potential anti-inflammatory steroidal Saponins from the berries of Solanum nigrum L. Journal of Agriculture Food and Chemistry. 2017;**65**:4262-4272

## Chapter 7

# Cryptorchidism in Pediatrics and Adults

*Shaban Memeti and Marijan Kamilovski*


## Abstract

Cryptorchidism, which is characterized by the failure of one or both testes to descend into the scrotum, presents unique challenges in both pediatric and adult populations. It is essential to provide early diagnosis and intervention in children, predominantly through orchiopexy, with laparoscopic assistance when required, to preserve fertility and reduce the risks of testicular atrophy and germ cell cancer. This chapter provides an in-depth classification of cryptorchidism, outlining its different types and their clinical significance. Cryptorchidism includes congenital forms like true undescended, ectopic, and retractile, as well as acquired ascending testis. It emphasizes the contributions of genetic, hormonal, and environmental factors. It emphasizes the contributions of genetic, hormonal, and environmental factors. Diagnostic techniques, including clinical examination, ultrasound, and diagnostic laparoscopy, as well as surgical and adjunct hormonal treatments, are discussed. In adults, cryptorchidism frequently goes undetected until complications appear, including malignancy, impaired spermatogenesis, or testicular atrophy. Management decisions involve weighing the benefits of orchiopexy against those of orchiectomy. The chapter highlights the significance of early detection, personalized treatment strategies, and long-term follow-up to optimize reproductive, oncologic, and psychosocial outcomes throughout the lifespan, emphasizing a multidisciplinary approach.


**Keywords:** cryptorchidism, undescended testis, orchiopexy, laparoscopy, testicular cancer, infertility, pediatric, and adult cryptorchidism

## 1. Introduction

Cryptorchidism, which is also referred to as undescended testes, is a congenital condition that is notably prevalent in male infants, particularly during the first year of life. Although the term may appear complex, its origins are straightforward: "crypto-" indicates hidden, and "orchid" implies testis, both of which are derived from the Greek language. The testes' fascinating voyage during fetal development is underscored by this condition, which frequently goes unnoticed until a clinical evaluation. This journey can occasionally pause or deviate from the anticipated course.

Cryptorchidism's unclear causes and long-term effects on hormonal function and fertility have puzzled scientists and clinicians for centuries. Despite advancements in surgical techniques and hormone-based treatments, many questions remain about the biological and environmental contributors to this condition.

Understanding cryptorchidism requires more than just medical terminology; it involves a detailed examination of the hormonal and anatomical mechanisms that regulate male fetal development.

This chapter delves into the biological origins of cryptorchidism and the most recent management strategies, explaining the significance of this condition for both health professionals and the general public [1].

## 2. Cryptorchidism in pediatrics

### 2.1 Definition of cryptorchidism

Cryptorchidism, or undescended testis, is the most prevalent congenital anomaly of the male reproductive system. It affects 2–5% of full-term neonates and is associated with hormonal dysfunction, fertility impairment, and an elevated risk of testicular malignancy [1]. Cryptorchidism, or undescended testis, is the most prevalent disorder of the male endocrine glands in infants, characterized by the absence of one or both testes from the dependent scrotum [2].

### 2.2 Embryology of cryptorchidism

Throughout the process of embryogenesis, the testes develop in proximity to the mesonephric kidneys and subsequently descend through the inguinal canal into the scrotal sac. There are three separate parts to this process: migration across the abdomen, development of the processus vaginalis and inguinal canal, and descent across the inguinal canal. The descent of the testicles is crucial for normal spermatogenesis, necessitating that the scrotal environment be maintained at a temperature 2–3°C lower than that of the body. A failure occurring during any stage of descent may lead to undescended testes (which remain stationary along the typical trajectory), ectopic testes (which deviate from the standard descent pathway), or absent testes (which may result from developmental failure or intrauterine loss). The gubernaculum, a mesenchymal structure, serves a vital function in securing and directing the descent of the testis. The process is regulated by hormonal mechanisms, wherein insulin-like factor 3 (INSL3) plays a crucial role in the initial masculinization and development of the gubernaculum, while testosterone governs the subsequent phase of gubernacular regression and the positioning of the scrotum. Cryptorchidism is linked to disruptions in hormonal signaling, notably in androgen receptor function, anti-Müllerian hormone (AMH) activity, and estrogen regulation. In addition, genetic factors such as SRY, SOX9, WT1, and SF1 play a key role in the development and descent of the testicles. In certain instances, cryptorchidism may be linked to congenital syndromes or environmental influences, including prenatal exposure to endocrine disruptors such as diethylstilbestrol (DES). Although the mechanisms regulating testicular descent have been thoroughly investigated, certain contentious aspects persist, particularly regarding the interaction between mechanical and hormonal influences [1].

### 2.3 Epidemiology

Cryptorchidism, typically diagnosed at birth as a congenital condition, can also be detected later in life [3]. Undescended testes affect 0.8% of boys at the age of one, increasing the risk of testicular germ cell cancer and germ cell deterioration by age two. Both undescended and contralateral testes are at risk for germ cell abnormalities, which can lead to infertility. Early orchiopexy before puberty reduces cancer incidence and improves spermatogenesis, shifting the focus from cancer risk to testicular function [4].

About 3% of full-term and 30% of preterm male newborns are born with one or both testicles undescended. Testicular descent typically occurs around the seventh month of gestation. However, over 80% of cryptorchid testes descend within the first 3 months of birth, lowering the true prevalence to about 1%. Cryptorchidism can occur unilaterally or bilaterally, with the right testicle being more commonly involved. Bilateral cryptorchidism occurs in around 10% of all patients with undescended testicles [5]. Prevalence rates exhibit significant regional variations, influenced by environmental, genetic, and socioeconomic factors [6].

Recent studies have reported prevalence rates of cryptorchidism ranging from 1 to 9% in full-term newborns. Notably, a comparative study observed a fourfold higher risk of cryptorchidism in Danish newborns (9.0%) compared to Finnish newborns (2.4%), after adjusting for confounders such as gestational age and birth weight. This variation underscores the influence of geographic and environmental factors on the incidence of cryptorchidism. Additionally, maternal smoking has been identified as a significant risk factor for the development of cryptorchidism [7].

### 2.4 Pathophysiology and etiology

The actual causes of cryptorchidism remain unknown. However, disturbances during the first and second phases of testicular descent can result in permanent failure. Testicular descent is a two-phase process regulated by hormones: the first phase occurs between 8 and 15 weeks, and the second between 25 and 35 weeks of gestation. The plausibility of a wide variety of potential risk factors in relation to the development of cryptorchidism remains debated. There are only a handful of factors that have consistent evidence of an association with cryptorchidism. When evidence is clear, the factor is often a proxy for the actual causative exposure. The importance of each risk factor may vary a lot between mother-son relationships because it depends on many genetic, maternal, placental, and fetal factors that can be different from one region to the next. Consequently, additional research is necessary to determine the role of causative factors in the etiology of cryptorchidism [8].

Cryptorchidism is a multifactorial condition. A normal hypothalamic-pituitary-gonadal axis is a prerequisite for testicular descent. Also, the body's structures must be able to interact with each other without being disturbed, and the right hormonal environment and environmental conditions must be present. Additionally, hereditary factors are significant. The Kaplan classification differentiates between palpable testes (80%) and nonpalpable testes (20%). There are testes that cannot be felt in three areas: the oblique, the inguinal, and the disappearing (vanishing) testes. Testes that can be felt are in the high scrotum, between the internal and external inguinal rings, or in a superficial pouch between the oblique and the Scarpa fascia [9].

Cryptorchidism is a complicated disorder with many causes. It happens when the testicles do not fall down properly during pregnancy. This process usually happens in two stages: transabdominal migration (8–15 weeks) and inguinoscrotal migration (25–35 weeks) [10]. Hormonal, genetic, environmental, and maternal factors that interfere with normal fetal development are to blame for testes not going down into the scrotum. Androgens and insulin-like factor 3 (INSL3) control the growth and migration of gubernacular cells through their receptors, which are called RXFP2 and AR, respectively. Cryptorchidism is linked to changes in the INSL3 gene because loss-of-function mutations in INSL3 or RXFP2 stop the development of the gonads and cause the testicles to not fall down properly [11–15].

Recent genetic research indicates that cryptorchidism is a multifactorial condition characterized by heterogeneous susceptibility. Genome-wide association studies (GWAS) have identified numerous loci that may be implicated in cryptorchidism, particularly those associated with cytoskeletal function and androgen receptor signaling pathways. Nonetheless, no individual genetic marker has been reliably replicated, suggesting a multifaceted genetic predisposition. The function of insulin-like factor 3 (INSL3) and its receptor LGR8 is essential in the process of testicular descent, as mutations in these genes have been associated with cryptorchidism in both animal and human research. INSL3 facilitates the development of the gubernaculum in a manner that is independent of androgens, whereas testosterone is accountable for the regression of the cranial suspensory ligament (CSL). Mutations in INSL3 have been linked to testicular dysgenesis syndrome (TDS), indicating a more extensive influence that extends beyond the process of testicular descent. Nevertheless, functional analyses of certain mutations do not consistently reveal modifications in INSL3 signaling, suggesting that other factors, including environmental influences, may play a role in the development of cryptorchidism [16–18].

Cryptorchidism is a multifactorial condition characterized by impaired androgen signaling, dysfunction of the gubernaculum, and genetic influences. Variants in the DHX37 gene indicate a potential involvement of impaired ribosomal function in testicular development, whereas elongated CAG and GGN repeats within the androgen receptor (AR) gene are associated with bilateral cryptorchidism. Mutations in INSL3, which are essential for the development of the gubernaculum, have been linked to testicular torsion, thereby underscoring its significance in the positioning of the testes. These findings underscore the heterogeneous etiology of cryptorchidism, which encompasses androgen resistance, gubernacular failure, and potential ribosomal defects [19–22].

## 2.5 Classification of cryptorchidism

Physical examinations categorize cryptorchidism into two categories: palpable testes and nonpalpable testes. Approximately 80% of cases present palpable testes, whereas 20% manifest with nonpalpable testes. The specific location of the testis plays a crucial role in determining clinical management strategies. Palpable testes encompass genuine undescended testes, ectopic testes, and retractile testes, the latter of which is frequently misdiagnosed as an undescended testis. Nonpalpable testes may be located intra-abdominally, within the inguinal canal, or may be entirely absent [1].

### *2.5.1 Palpable testes*

#### *2.5.1.1 Undescended testis*

A true undescended testis is one that has halted along the normal descent path. Its palpability may vary based on its location. Inguinal testes, for instance, may have ceased their descent within the inguinal canal; however, they are not always noticeable upon physical examination. When examined laparoscopically, certain testes may be identified as “peeping” testes, indicating that they intermittently traverse in and out of the internal inguinal ring. When the testes are raised, the spermatic vessels get smaller, there are problems with the Wolffian duct, and there are more cases of inguinal hernia [23].

##### *2.5.1.2 Ectopic testis*

An ectopic testis diverges from its normal descent trajectory and may be located at atypical sites, such as the superficial inguinal pouch, perineum, femoral region, or penile shaft, or it may even migrate to the contralateral inguinal canal [24].

##### *2.5.1.3 Retractile testis*

A typical form in which the testis is not initially located in the lower scrotum but can be painlessly maneuvered into a low scrotal location, where it subsequently remains [25].

#### *2.5.2 Nonpalpable testes*

##### *2.5.2.1 Intra-abdominal testes*

An intra-abdominal testis is a form of undescended testis located within the abdominal cavity, accounting for approximately 5% of all undescended testes. This condition is associated with increased risks of infertility and testicular malignancy. Early surgical intervention, typically before 1 year of age, is recommended to mitigate these risks. Laparoscopy is commonly employed for both diagnosis and treatment, with the two-stage Fowler-Stephens procedure being a preferred surgical approach due to its favorable outcomes [25–27].

##### *2.5.2.2 Absent testes (vanishing testis syndrome)*

The testis is absent, potentially due to agenesis or atrophy caused by intrauterine occurrences such as testicular torsion or vascular incidents [28].

##### *2.5.2.3 Testicular agenesis*

Testicular agenesis, or congenital absence of the testis, is an uncommon disorder characterized by the absence of one or both testes at birth. A research examining instances of nonpalpable testes revealed that roughly 27% of cases of absent testes were due to full agenesis, characterized by the absence of both the testis and related structures such as the epididymis and vas deferens [29].

#### *2.5.3 Bilateral undescended testes*

Bilateral cryptorchidism occurs when both testes fail to descend into the scrotum before birth. This disease occurs in roughly 1% of male infants at the age of 1 year.

Early identification and intervention are essential, as bilateral undescended testes correlate with an increased risk of infertility and testicular malignancy. Surgical intervention, generally conducted between 6 months and 2 years of age, is advised to relocate the testes into the scrotum [30, 31].

### *2.5.3.1 Clinical significance*

The precise classification of cryptorchidism is crucial for the formulation of appropriate treatment strategies. Palpable testes may necessitate only monitoring or minor surgical repositioning, whereas nonpalpable testes require advanced imaging techniques or laparoscopic intervention. Furthermore, differentiating among retractile, ascending, and ectopic testes is essential in averting unwarranted surgical procedures and facilitating prompt intervention, thereby mitigating the risk of long-term complications such as subfertility and testicular malignancy [1].

## 2.6 Clinical presentation and diagnosis

Cryptorchidism, or undescended testis, is the most common congenital genitourinary disorder in male neonates, affecting approximately 1–2% of boys older than 6 months. While spontaneous descent often occurs within the first 3 months of life, the likelihood of further descent after 6 months is low, necessitating timely evaluation and management. Clinical diagnosis is primarily based on a thorough history and physical examination. Factors such as prematurity, intrauterine growth restriction, and family history of cryptorchidism should be assessed, given their association with the condition.

A key clinical finding is the absence of one or both testes from the scrotum. Testes may be palpable or nonpalpable, with the latter requiring further assessment to distinguish intra-abdominal testis, atrophic testis, or testicular agenesis. A distinction must also be made between true undescended testes, which fail to descend along the normal path, and retractile testes, which are mobile and can be manipulated into the scrotum. Retractile testes, influenced by an exaggerated cremasteric reflex, are typically benign and rarely necessitate surgical intervention, except in cases of progressive ascent.

The majority of cryptorchid testes are palpable and are commonly located in the inguinal canal, near the external inguinal ring, or just above the scrotum. The presence of an inguinal mass may lead to misdiagnosis as an inguinal hernia, necessitating careful differentiation. In contrast, nonpalpable testes occur in approximately 20% of cases and pose a greater diagnostic challenge. Laparoscopy is the preferred modality for localization of nonpalpable testes, as imaging techniques such as ultrasound and MRI have limited accuracy and do not significantly alter management. Meta-analyses have demonstrated that ultrasound has a sensitivity of 45% and specificity of 78% in detecting nonpalpable testes, making it an unreliable diagnostic tool.

International guidelines emphasize the importance of early referral to a surgical specialist if the testes have not descended by 6 months of age. Early orchiopexy, ideally performed between 6 and 18 months, optimizes fertility potential and reduces the risk of testicular malignancy. Patients with bilateral cryptorchidism or suspected disorders of sex development require additional endocrinologic and genetic evaluation to exclude conditions such as hypogonadotropic hypogonadism or androgen insensitivity syndrome.

Bilateral nonpalpable testes necessitate a hormonal workup, including measurement of anti-Müllerian hormone (AMH) and stimulated testosterone response to human chorionic gonadotropin (hCG). A lack of testosterone rise suggests testicular agenesis or anorchia. Patients with unilateral cryptorchidism have an infertility rate of up to 10%, while those with bilateral undescended testes or delayed orchiopexy have significantly higher infertility risks. Testicular cancer risk is also elevated, with a threefold increase compared to the general population, necessitating lifelong testicular self-examination after puberty [32–37]. **Figure 1**: Comparative imaging modalities in cryptorchidism. The upper image shows a coronal view of an MRI, highlighting undescended testes with clear soft tissue differentiation. The lower image displays a 3D CT reconstruction, illustrating anatomical relations and vascular structures. MRI is preferred for its superior soft tissue contrast, while CT may be used in selected cases for detailed anatomical visualization, particularly when assessing vascular anomalies or planning surgical intervention.

### *2.6.1 Clinical examination*

The clinical examination of cryptorchidism is essential for determining the testicular position and guiding management. It should be performed in a warm environment to minimize the cremasteric reflex, which can cause retraction. The examination begins with inspection of the scrotum for asymmetry or underdevelopment, followed by palpation along the testicular descent path, including the inguinal canal and perineum. A retractile testis, which can be manipulated into the scrotum and remains there, is benign and requires no treatment, whereas a true undescended

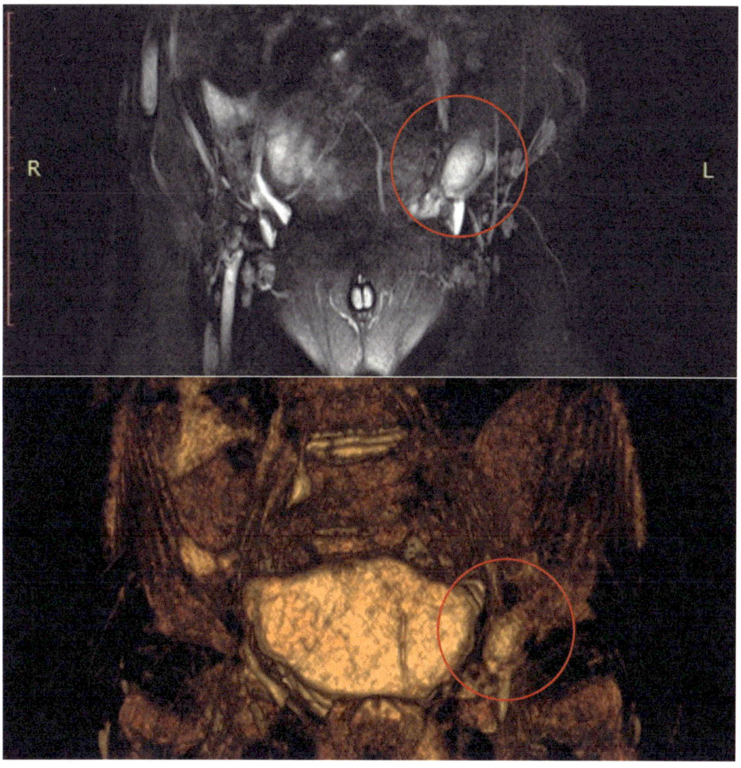


**Figure 1.**
*Compares imaging modalities for cryptorchidism. The upper image shows a coronal view of an MRI, which shows undescended testes with distinct soft tissue differentiation. The lower image shows a 3D CT reconstruction that illustrates anatomical relationships and circulatory systems. MRI is recommended due to its superior soft tissue contrast, although CT can be employed in certain circumstances for comprehensive anatomical visualization, notably when assessing vascular abnormalities or planning surgical intervention.*

testis cannot be manually positioned in the scrotum. Approximately 80% of undescended testes are palpable and localized in the inguinal region, near the external inguinal ring, or prescrotally, while nonpalpable cases may be intra-abdominal, atrophic, or absent. The contralateral testis should be checked for hypertrophy, which suggests testicular agenesis or regression. Specialized maneuvers such as the milking maneuver help differentiate an inguinal hernia from an undescended testis, while the absence of the cremasteric reflex may indicate a high testicular position. In nonpalpable cases, further assessment with laparoscopy is often required, as imaging techniques like ultrasound and MRI have limited accuracy. Hormonal tests, including AMH and hCG stimulation, may be useful in bilateral cases to assess testicular function and exclude disorders of sex development. Early diagnosis and timely orchiopexy between 6 and 18 months are crucial for preserving fertility potential and reducing the risk of testicular cancer [33, 34, 37]. Physical examination is still the primary method for diagnosing cryptorchidism. As seen in the photographs in **Figure 2**, the examination entails palpating the inguinal canal and scrotum in order to find and mobilize the testis. Positioning the child comfortably, such as with the leg slightly abducted and externally rotated, relaxes the cremasteric reflex and increases the possibility of finding a retractile or undescended testis. This approach distinguishes real undescended testes from retractile or ectopic testes, allowing for more precise diagnosis and care planning.

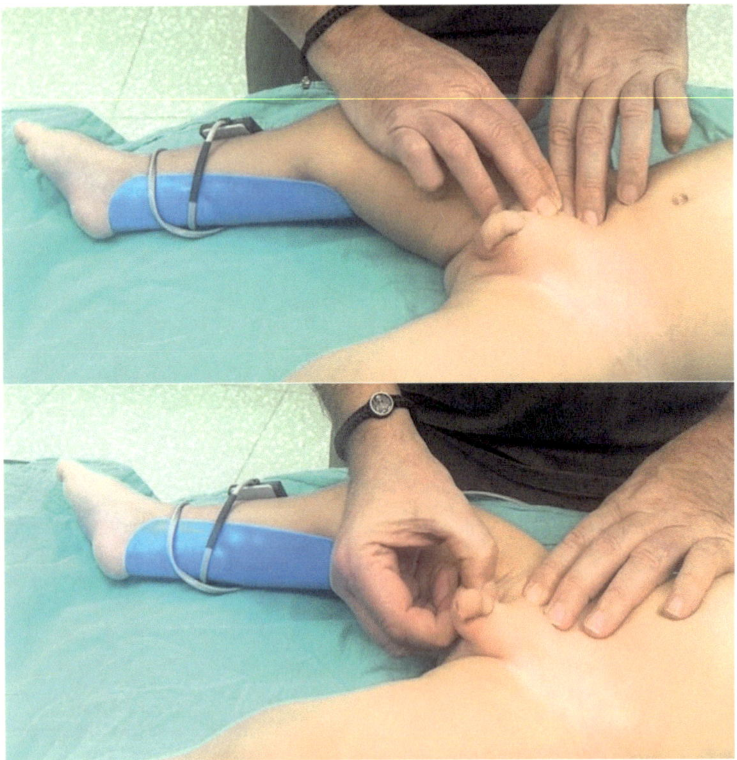

**Figure 2.**
*Illustrates physical examination approaches for cryptorchidism. The upper image shows palpation of the inguinal region to identify a potentially undescended testis, while the lower image shows mild manipulation to check testicular mobility and probable displacement inside the scrotum. Proper placement of the child and a comfortable setting are critical for reducing the cremasteric reaction during the examination.*

### 2.6.2 Ultrasound and Doppler imaging

Ultrasound is frequently used in the diagnosis of nonpalpable cryptorchidism, although its clinical value is limited. According to studies, ultrasound has a sensitivity of around 45% and a specificity of 78% in detecting intra-abdominal testes, making it unreliable for conclusive localization. Its capacity to distinguish between a missing, atrophic, or intra-abdominal testis is limited, frequently resulting in wasteful imaging and increased healthcare expenses without appreciably affecting management. While ultrasonography may help find inguinal testes and guide surgical procedures, laparoscopy remains the gold standard for diagnosing and treating nonpalpable testes. Inguinal ultrasonography, when paired with an assessment of contralateral testicular enlargement, can increase the accuracy of deciding whether an inguinal or laparoscopic approach is required, potentially resulting in fewer needless surgeries. However, worldwide guidelines prohibit the routine use of ultrasound in the diagnosis of undescended testes because it does not significantly help decision-making and should not cause a delay in surgical referral [34–36]. As seen in the photographs in **Figure 3**, ultrasonography allows for visibility of the testis within the inguinal canal, providing information on its size, echogenicity, and vascularity. This imaging

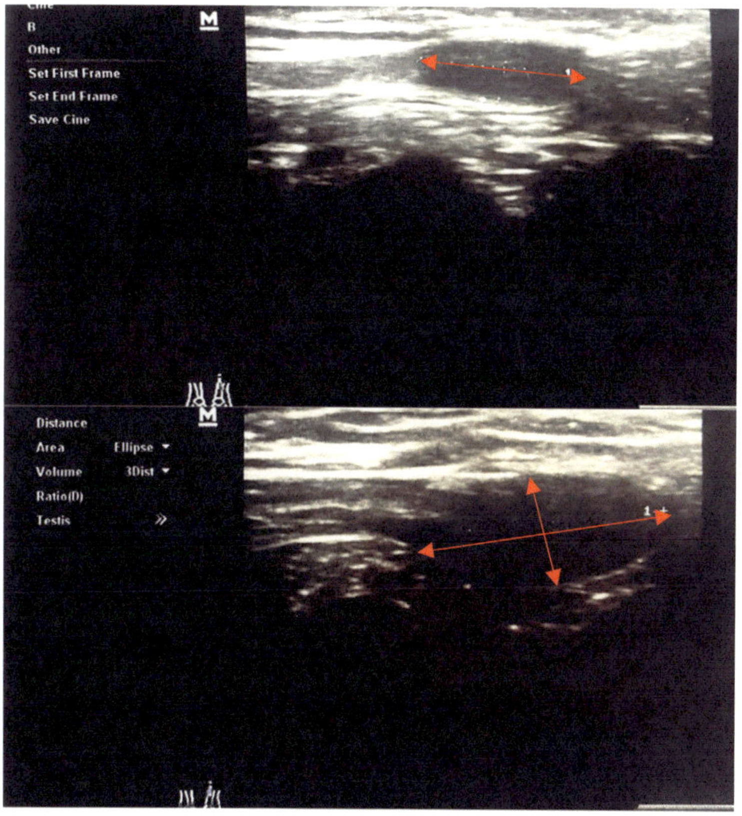


**Figure 3.**
*Shows ultrasound imaging of cryptorchidism. The upper image shows the inguinal area, which includes an undescended testis with a hypoechoic structure. The lower image shows a closer look at the testicular parenchyma, which confirms the presence and size of the testis within the inguinal canal.*

technique helps to differentiate undescended testes from other diseases, such as atrophic or nonexistent testes, directing subsequent care and surgical planning.

*2.6.3 Laparoscopy*

Laparoscopy is an effective diagnostic and therapeutic method for managing impalpable testes, providing both localization and treatment choices. A classification system based on laparoscopic results can help guide surgical decisions. Testes can be classified into four types: missing, internal ring with looping vessels, internal ring with direct vessel entry, and intra-abdominal. Depending on the testicular position and vascular anatomy, therapeutic options include one-stage laparoscopic orchiopexy, phased orchiopexy after vessel ligation, or testicular excision if atrophy occurs. Laparoscopic-assisted orchiopexy is the preferred treatment for managing nonpalpable testes due to its efficacy and low risk of testicular atrophy and retraction [38].

## 2.7 Surgical intervention and management

The primary goal of cryptorchidism treatment in pediatric patients is to relocate the undescended testis into the scrotum prior to the age of 18 months in order to reduce the risk of long-term complications, including infertility, testicular atrophy, and malignancy.

*2.7.1 Orchiopexy (surgical intervention)*

Orchiopexy is the gold-standard surgical intervention for cryptorchidism, involving the repositioning of the undescended testis into the scrotum to optimize fertility and reduce oncologic risks. The procedure entails transferring the testicle from its aberrant location—usually within the belly or groin—into the scrotum and anchoring it in place. To achieve the best results, this treatment is often indicated for infants aged 6 to 18 months. Early management is critical since untreated undescended testicles are associated with an increased risk of infertility and testicular cancer later in life. Orchiopexy has a high success rate, with studies showing that the procedure is approximately 100% effective at appropriately positioning the testicle within the scrotum. The operation is typically performed as an outpatient under general anesthesia, which allows for a speedy recovery. Postoperative treatment includes monitoring for problems such as infection or testicular atrophy, which are infrequent. Timely orchiopexy not only improves fertility and lowers the chance of cancer, but it also makes it easier to examine the testicles for any future anomalies [39].

*2.7.2 Laparoscopy*

Because of its diagnostic and therapeutic benefits, laparoscopic orchiopexy has emerged as the primary method for managing nonpalpable and intra-abdominal testes. Laparoscopy provides direct vision of the testis, spermatic arteries, and vas deferens, allowing for more informed surgical decisions. The Fowler-Stephens procedure is still the gold standard for high intra-abdominal testes, with both one-stage and two-stage approaches achieving success rates of 80–91%. The two-stage treatment, which involves ligating spermatic arteries first and then performing delayed orchiopexy, has been linked to improved testicular survival by allowing for the formation of collateral blood supplies. Emerging treatments, including gubernaculum-sparing laparoscopic orchiopexy and the Shehata traction technique, seek to increase testicular vitality and decrease atrophy rates. While laparoscopic orchiopexy has demonstrated efficacy, long-term studies are required to establish its effects on reproductive results [40]. **Figure 4** highlights the main surgical phases and provides a step-by-step illustration of orchiopexy for cryptorchidism. This procedure substantially reduces the risk of infertility and testicular malignancy.

Recent advancements have led to the development of in vitro models that predict patient responses to human chorionic gonadotropin (hCG) therapy. By cultivating and treating primary cells derived from cryptorchid patients' gubernaculum testis biopsies, researchers can analyze the effects of hCG on cell proliferation and differentiation. This approach enables the tailoring of adjuvant therapies to individual patients, potentially improving outcomes and reducing unnecessary treatments [41].

### *2.7.3 Complications of orchiopexy*

Orchiopexy is the standard surgical intervention for cryptorchidism. Although it is generally considered safe, it is associated with potential complications. The primary risk of considerable concern is testicular atrophy, which may arise as a consequence of:

Surgical procedures can cause damage to the spermatic vessels.

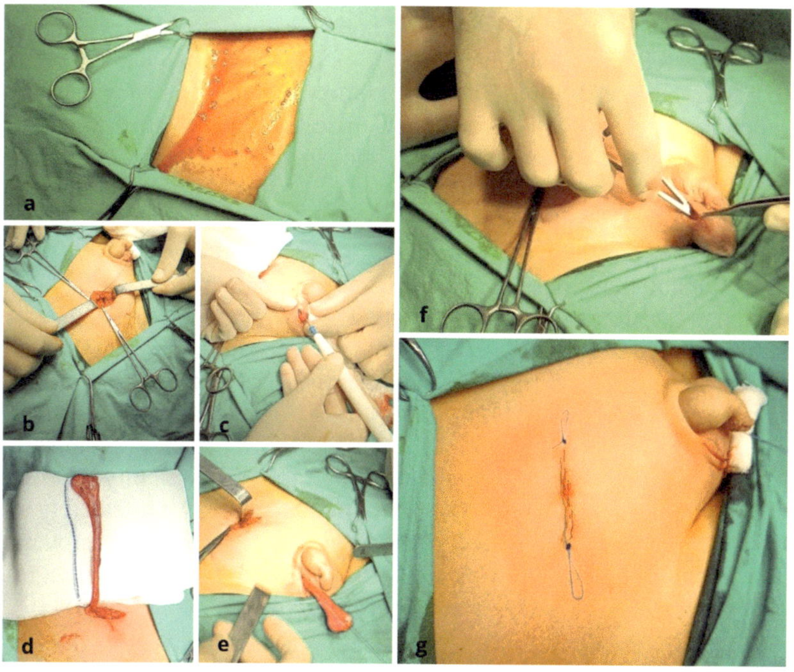


**Figure 4.**
*The surgical correction of cryptorchidism is illustrated in sequential phases. After preparing the surgical field under sterile conditions, an incision is made in the inguinal region to expose the inguinal canal (1a). The inguinal canal is dissected and retracted to visualize the undescended testis (1b). The testis and spermatic cord are mobilized by carefully dividing the cremasteric fibers and freeing them from surrounding adhesions while maintaining hemostasis (1c). Any associated hernia sac is identified, isolated, ligated, and reduced to prevent the recurrence of an inguinal hernia (1d). A scrotal pouch is created to accommodate the testis, which is then passed through a subcutaneous tunnel into the scrotum (1e). The testis is fixed securely in place using sutures to prevent torsion and maintain its position within the scrotum (1f). Finally, the surgical site is closed in layers, ensuring proper alignment and minimal scarring (1 g).*

Tension exerted on the spermatic vessels results in ischemia.

Unintentional torsion of the spermatic vessels may occur during the placement of the testis within the scrotum.

The procedure involves the intentional ligation of the spermatic vessels during Fowler-Stephens orchidopexy.

Furthermore, complications that are frequently encountered in the repair of inguinal hernias may similarly occur during the procedure of orchiopexy. Testicular retraction may arise from several factors, including shortened testicular vessels, insufficient mobilization of the vascular pedicle, incomplete severance of the cremasteric muscle fibers, or inadequate fixation of the testis within the scrotum. While infrequent, these complications underscore the necessity of meticulous surgical technique and vigilant postoperative monitoring to guarantee optimal outcomes [1].

## 2.8 Complications and long-term outcomes

### *2.8.1 Testicular cancer*

Cryptorchidism is a well-known risk factor for testicular cancer, with affected individuals having a three to eightfold higher risk than the general population. The danger is greatest for intra-abdominal testes and situations when orchiopexy is delayed past puberty. Germ cell tumors, notably seminomas, are the most prevalent cancers linked with undescended testes, but non-seminomatous germ cell tumors can also occur. Early orchiopexy, ideally before 12–18 months of age, has been demonstrated to lessen, but not eliminate, this risk. Individuals with a history of cryptorchidism should undergo long-term surveillance, including self-examination and clinical follow-ups, in order to allow early detection and treatment of testicular cancer [40].

### *2.8.2 Testicular torsion*

Testicular torsion is a serious complication associated with cryptorchidism, occurring due to the abnormal fixation of the testis, which predisposes it to twisting around the spermatic cord. This leads to vascular compromise, causing ischemia and potential testicular necrosis if not treated promptly. Cryptorchid testes, particularly those located intra-abdominally or in the inguinal canal, are at a higher risk of torsion due to the absence of normal scrotal fixation. The clinical presentation includes acute scrotal pain, swelling, nausea, and vomiting, with rapid progression to infarction if not treated within 6–8 hours. Surgical intervention is required immediately to untwist and fixate the testis or, in severe cases, perform orchiectomy. Early orchiopexy reduces the risk of torsion by securing the testis within the scrotum, highlighting the importance of timely surgical correction in cryptorchidism management [40].

### *2.8.3 Inguinal hernia*

The medical literature clearly establishes a link between inguinal hernia and cryptorchidism. Cryptorchidism is commonly accompanied by a patent processus vaginalis, an embryologic remnant that allows the testes to descend. When this structure fails to shut, the individual is more likely to develop an indirect inguinal hernia. According to studies, more than 90% of cryptorchidism individuals may have an inguinal hernia, especially if the testis remains within the inguinal canal. The occurrence of an inguinal hernia in cryptorchid patients emphasizes the importance of timely surgical correction (orchiopexy) to avoid consequences such as hernia incarceration, testicular torsion, and infertility [23].

#### *2.8.4 Hypogonadism and impaired fertility*

Cryptorchidism is a well-established risk factor for hypogonadism and impaired fertility, with both unilateral and bilateral cases contributing to long-term reproductive consequences. The failure of testicular descent results in prolonged exposure of the testes to intra-abdominal temperatures, which disrupts normal spermatogenesis and Leydig cell function. As a consequence, patients with untreated bilateral cryptorchidism frequently develop azoospermia, with studies indicating that up to 98% of these individuals are infertile. Even in cases of unilateral cryptorchidism, there is a significant reduction in sperm count and quality due to the adverse impact on the contralateral descended testis, likely influenced by shared intrinsic pathology.

Surgical intervention, especially orchiopexy, preserves fertility. Early correction, especially before 1 year, enhances testicular function and adult spermatogenesis, according to research. Childhood orchiopexy reduces azoospermia to 32% in bilateral instances and 46% in unilateral cryptorchidism, lowering the likelihood of infertility. After successful repositioning, these patients are at risk of subfertility and endocrine dysfunction, therefore long-term follow-up is necessary. Cryptorchidism causes adult hypogonadism due to testosterone deficiency and poor spermatogenesis. Defective Leydig cell function, especially bilaterally, can lower testosterone levels, causing delayed puberty, diminished secondary sexual characteristics, and metabolic issues. Although hormone therapy has been studied as an adjuvant to surgery, current fertility recommendations recommend early orchiopexy. Cryptorchidism increases the incidence of testicular germ cell cancers, emphasizing the need for early identification and treatment [42, 43].

Emerging evidence suggests that epigenetic modifications play a significant role in the infertility risk associated with cryptorchidism. Cryptorchid boys with defective mini-puberty and impaired differentiation of Ad spermatogonia exhibit altered expression of genes encoding histone methyltransferases. These epigenetic changes may contribute to impaired spermatogenesis and increased infertility risk [44].

#### *2.8.5 Testicular atrophy*

Testicular atrophy is a serious long-term complication of cryptorchidism, caused by prolonged exposure of the undescended testis to an aberrant intra-abdominal or inguinal environment. Elevated temperature, poor vascular supply, and intrinsic testicular dysgenesis all lead to progressive germ cell loss and Leydig cell failure. Histological studies show that atrophic testes have reduced spermatogonia, poor Sertoli cell growth, and increased fibrosis, resulting in irreparable damage and an increased chance of infertility.

Early orchiopexy, preferably before 12 months of age, significantly reduces the risk of testicular atrophy and optimizes spermatogenesis. However, delaying surgical intervention considerably raises the risk of testicular atrophy and poor spermatogenesis. According to studies, testicular atrophy rates after orchiopexy range from 5 to 32%, with greater rates found in cases with intra-abdominal testes that require phased treatments. Furthermore, testicular atrophy is more likely in individuals following Fowler-Stephens orchiopexy due to the need for spermatic artery closure, which reduces testicular blood flow.

Despite surgical intervention, atrophic testes may still produce insufficient testosterone, predisposing affected persons to hypogonadism and infertility. Patients with a history of cryptorchidism require long-term follow-up to check testicular volume, endocrine function, and reproductive potential [40, 45, 46].

## 3. Cryptorchidism in adults

### 3.1 Definition of cryptorchidism

Cryptorchidism, also known as undescended testicles (UDTs), is uncommon in adult males, and even less often when it occurs bilaterally. While pediatric management is well established, guidelines for adult cryptorchidism remain less defined, with debates over the benefits of late orchiopexy versus orchidectomy [47].

### 3.2 Epidemiology

While cryptorchidism is commonly diagnosed and treated in infancy, a significant number of cases remain undetected until adolescence or adulthood, particularly in developing countries where healthcare access may be limited. Studies indicate that approximately 21% of cryptorchid patients undergoing surgery are 12 years or older, with a mean age of 25.4 years, and some cases reported even in the fourth decade of life. The condition predominantly presents as unilateral cryptorchidism, with the right side affected more frequently, though bilateral undescended testes occur in about 17% of cases. The delayed diagnosis raises concerns due to increased risks of infertility, hypogonadism, and testicular malignancy, yet there remains significant variation in surgical management, with many adult cases undergoing orchidopexy rather than orchidectomy, despite guideline recommendations for testicular removal in post-pubertal patients [48].

Early recognition and surgical repair before 1 year of age are crucial to reduce the negative impact of both unilateral and bilateral cryptorchidism. The timing of surgery is associated with better testicular volume and spermatogenic outcomes. Regarding surgical techniques, the choice between one-stage and two-stage orchiopexy for intra-abdominal testes remains debated. The Fowler-Stephens (FS) staged approach, which involves ligation of spermatic vessels, has documented success rates between 80 and 86%. Alternative methodologies, such as the Shehata technique, emphasize traction-induced elongation to optimize vascular preservation and achieve sufficient mobilization [40].

### 3.3 Clinical presentation in adults

In adult patients, cryptorchidism is sometimes identified accidentally during clinical assessments for infertility, scrotal asymmetry, or testicular pain. The undescended testis is generally smaller than the contralateral testis and is often palpable, with the inguinal region being the predominant site. In a study of adult cryptorchidism, 82.4% of unilateral patients and all bilateral cases exhibited a palpable testis, while a lesser proportion presented with prepubic or intra-abdominal testes. Histological analysis often uncovers anatomical anomalies like testicular atrophy, hypospermatogenesis, and Sertoli cell-only syndrome, indicative of compromised spermatogenesis and testicular dysfunction. Semen analysis frequently reveals impaired fertility, with results including azoospermia and asthenozoospermia. The fact that cryptorchidism is not always diagnosed and treated until adulthood shows how important regular medical exams are, especially for people who are having trouble getting pregnant or have strange problems with their testicles [49].

Adult patients with unilateral cryptorchidism frequently exhibit a modest clinical picture that conceals severe underlying histological and functional changes. Many individuals, who are often diagnosed in early adulthood, may be asymptomatic in terms of fertility, with a tendency toward normospermia, especially if the undescended testis has a bigger volume. People with smaller testicles, on the other hand, often have abnormal semen parameters like azoospermia or oligo−/asthenospermia. This shows that there is a strong link between smaller testicles and problems with spermatogenesis. Importantly, routine physical examinations and imaging modalities may not reliably predict the underlying pathology, as there is no significant relationship between testicular localization (intra-abdominal, within the inguinal canal, or in the superficial inguinal region) and histopathological outcomes. A close look at the tissue often shows signs like Sertoli cell-only syndrome, testicular shrinkage, or even a testis that is missing (anorchia), which means that the germ cells will be affected negatively in the long term. Endocrine function, which is mostly kept up by Leydig cells, may slowly decline over time, but this does not seem to have a big effect on fertility, and germ cell cancers are not usually found by accident. There is a big difference between having mild symptoms and having small but noticeable changes in the tissue. This raises important questions about when and if an orchiectomy is necessary for adults with unilateral cryptorchidism versus conservative management [50].

Adult cryptorchidism is frequently diagnosed incidentally during medical evaluations for infertility, scrotal asymmetry, or testicular discomfort. Many cases remain undiagnosed due to the lack of symptoms, while others present with nonspecific complaints such as groin pain or reduced testicular volume. In a study analyzing adult cryptorchid patients, hormonal profiling revealed lower serum testosterone and inhibin B levels, indicating impaired Leydig and Sertoli cell function. Moreover, approximately 40–50% of adult patients with untreated cryptorchidism exhibit semen abnormalities, including azoospermia or severe oligozoospermia, affecting fertility outcomes [51].

Additionally, cryptorchid testes in adults are often atrophic, fibrotic, and display histopathological changes suggestive of germ cell neoplasia in situ (GCNIS), reinforcing the need for timely intervention. The lack of descent results in prolonged exposure to intra-abdominal temperatures, causing irreversible damage to spermatogenesis and hormone production [52].

### 3.4 Surgical intervention in adults

Orchiopexy is the main surgery used to treat cryptorchidism in adults. This procedure involves moving and securing the undescended testis inside the scrotum.

The location of the testis determines the surgical strategy. Testes that are palpable in the inguinal canal undergo an open inguinal orchiopexy. This procedure entails making an inguinal incision to access and move the testis, which is then fixed within the scrotum. This method lets you see the spermatic cord clearly and carefully cut it, which keeps the testicular function and reduces damage to the blood vessels [50].

Diagnostic laparoscopy is the initial step in locating a nonpalpable testis. If an orchiopexy is discovered in the belly, a laparoscopic method is used, resulting in less postoperative pain and a faster recovery. If the testis is positioned high intra-abdominally and has a short vascular pedicle, a two-stage Fowler-Stephens orchiopexy is recommended. This treatment begins with the ligation of the testicular arteries to stimulate collateral circulation, followed by a second stage of surgery to relocate the testis in the scrotum.

Orchiectomy (testicular removal) is advised when the testis is atrophic or there is a high risk of cancer. This is especially important in older people whose fertility is already limited or when testicular cancer is suspected based on ultrasonographic abnormalities or tumor markers [53].

The decision to perform orchiopexy versus orchiectomy in adult cryptorchid patients remains a topic of clinical debate. Orchiectomy is generally recommended for intra-abdominal testes, particularly if atrophic or associated with histological abnormalities, due to the increased malignancy risk. However, for palpable inguinal testes with preserved structure, orchiopexy remains an option, particularly in younger adults wishing to preserve hormonal function [54].

Recent advancements in laparoscopic and robotic-assisted orchiopexy have improved outcomes for adult patients. Robotic-assisted orchiopexy has shown advantages in precision and reduced recovery time, particularly for intra-abdominal testes, and is increasingly used in specialized centers [54, 55]. A meta-analysis comparing open versus laparoscopic orchiopexy in adults found that laparoscopic approaches were associated with lower postoperative pain, shorter hospital stays, and improved testicular viability. Furthermore, testicular repositioning before the age of 30 is associated with better long-term testosterone production [56].

### 3.5 Associated risks in adults

Cryptorchidism in adults is a rare but clinically significant condition that poses increased risks of infertility, endocrine dysfunction, and testicular malignancy. Late diagnosis often results in irreversible histopathological changes, including spermatogenic failure and Leydig cell dysfunction, which can lead to reduced testosterone levels and metabolic disturbances. Management strategies depend on the testicular position, viability, and malignancy risk. While orchiectomy is commonly recommended for atrophic or intra-abdominal testes, laparoscopic and robotic-assisted orchiopexy remain viable options for preserving hormonal function and preventing further complications. Recent studies highlight the efficacy of minimally invasive approaches in adults, demonstrating lower postoperative morbidity and improved testicular outcomes [48, 55, 57].

#### *3.5.1 Testicular cancer*

Men with a history of cryptorchidism, especially those with untreated or undescended testes, are more likely to develop testicular cancer [58]. The higher risk may be because of the abnormal temperature and hormonal environment of the testis that has not descended. This makes the tissue more likely to develop genetic problems and turn cancerous [59].

#### *3.5.2 Infertility*

Cryptorchidism can lead to infertility, which is caused by poor spermatogenesis in the undescended testis [60]. The aberrant anatomical location exposes the testicular tissue to temperatures over the acceptable range, disrupting the delicate process of sperm generation. Histopathological investigations usually indicate abnormalities—such as Sertoli cell-only syndrome, maturation arrest, or testicular atrophy—which are associated with low sperm counts and poor fertility [61].

### *3.5.3 Psychosocial effects*

Psychosocial pressures can impact interpersonal relationships as well as overall mental health, emphasizing the importance of a multidisciplinary strategy that includes psychological treatment and support [62].

## 4. Conclusion

Cryptorchidism is a complex condition that necessitates early detection, prompt care, and long-term monitoring to improve fertility, oncologic outcomes, and psychosocial well-being. Approximately 2–5% of full-term babies are born with this condition. Its cause is complicated and includes genetic, hormonal, environmental, and epigenetic factors. While spontaneous testicular descent occurs within the first 6 months of birth, chronic cryptorchidism requires surgical treatment to reduce the risks of infertility, testicular atrophy, and cancer. Orchiopexy performed before 12 months of age is the current standard of care, offering the greatest benefits in fertility preservation and malignancy risk reduction.

While hormone therapy is still contentious, increasing research suggests it may have a role in postoperative fertility enhancement, particularly for bilateral cryptorchidism.

Cryptorchidism is usually detected inadvertently in adults as a result of infertility, scrotal asymmetry, or testicular pain. The choice between orchiopexy and orchiectomy is determined by criteria such as testicular atrophy, cancer risk, and patient preferences. Adult patients frequently necessitate oncologic surveillance due to the much greater incidence of testicular germ cell cancers. Furthermore, psychosocial distress, such as anxiety, sadness, and body image issues, needs integrated mental health care to improve quality of life.

## Acknowledgements

The authors wish to extend their heartfelt appreciation to Dr. Haris Sulejmani, MD, for his significant support and perceptive input during the creation of this chapter. His proficiency, commitment, and scrupulous attention to detail have significantly enhanced the substance and clarity of our work. We much value his assistance in enhancing the manuscript and guaranteeing its scholarly integrity.

## Conflict of interest

The authors declare no conflict of interest.

## Acronyms and abbreviations

| | |
|---|---|
| AMH | anti-Müllerian hormone |
| AUA | American Urological Association |

| | |
|---|---|
| CAH | congenital adrenal hyperplasia |
| CIS | carcinoma in situ |
| CUA | Canadian Urological Association |
| DES | diethylstilbestrol |
| EDCs | endocrine-disrupting chemicals |
| EAU | European Association of Urology |
| FSO | Fowler-Stephens Orchiopexy |
| FSH | follicle-stimulating hormone |
| GWAS | Genome-Wide Association Study |
| hCG | human chorionic gonadotropin |
| INSL3 | insulin-like factor 3 |
| LH | luteinizing hormone |
| LHRH | luteinizing hormone-releasing hormone |
| MIS | Müllerian Inhibiting Substance |
| MRI | magnetic resonance imaging |
| NR5A1 | Nuclear Receptor Subfamily 5 Group A Member 1 |
| RXFP2 | relaxin/insulin-like family peptide receptor 2 |
| SF1 | steroidogenic factor 1 |
| SRY | sex-determining region Y |
| TAI | testicular atrophy index |
| TGFBR3 | transforming growth factor beta receptor 3 |
| TV | testicular volume |
| UDT | undescended testis |
| US | ultrasound |
| WT1 | Wilms' tumor 1 |

*DOI: http://dx.doi.org/10.5772/intechopen.1010262*

## Author details

Shaban Memeti* and Marijan Kamilovski
University Clinic of Pediatric Surgery, Skopje, North Macedonia

*Address all correspondence to: shab28me@yahoo.com

## References

[1] Gearhart JP, Rink RC, Mouriquand PDE. Pediatric Urology. 2nd ed. Philadelphia, PA: Saunders; 2010

[2] Greenfield SP, Cooper CS. Pediatric Urology for Primary Care. Elk Grove Village, IL: American Academy of Pediatrics Publishing Staff; 2019

[3] Partin AW, Dmochowski RR, Kavoussi LR, Peters CA. Campbell Walsh Wein Urology. 12th ed. S.L.: Elsevier; 2020

[4] Mcaninch JW, Lue TF. Smith and Tanagho's General Urology. 19th ed. New York: McGraw-Hill Education; 2020

[5] Leslie SW, Sajjad H, Villanueva CA. Cryptorchidism [Internet]. Treasure Island (FL): StatPearls Publishing; 2024. Available from: https://www.ncbi.nlm.nih.gov/books/NBK470270/

[6] Kollin C, Ritzén EM. Cryptorchidism: A clinical perspective. Pediatric Endocrinology Reviews: PER [Internet]. 2014;**11**(Suppl. 2):240-250. Available from: https://pubmed.ncbi.nlm.nih.gov/24683948/

[7] Holmboe SA, Beck AL, Andersson AM, Main KM, Jørgensen N, Skakkebæk NE, et al. The epidemiology of cryptorchidism and potential risk factors, including endocrine disrupting chemicals. Frontiers in Endocrinology [Internet]. 2024;**15**:15. Available from: https://www.ncbi.nlm.nih.gov/pmc/articles/PMC11021654/#B37

[8] Gurney JK, McGlynn KA, Stanley J, Merriman T, Signal V, Shaw C, et al. Risk factors for cryptorchidism. Nature Reviews Urology [Internet]. 2017;**14**(9):534-548. Available from: https://www.nature.com/articles/nrurol.2017.90?draft=collection

[9] Comploj E, Pycha A. Diagnosis and management of cryptorchidism. European Urology Supplements. 2012;**11**(2):2-9

[10] 9.Boisen K, Kaleva M, Main K, Virtanen H, Haavisto A-M, Schmidt I, et al. Difference in prevalence of congenital cryptorchidism in infants between two Nordic countries. The Lancet. 2004;**363**(9417):1264

[11] Hutson JM, Li R, Southwell BR, Newgreen D, Cousinery M. Regulation of testicular descent. Pediatric Surgery International. 2015;**31**(4):317-325

[12] Bay K, Main KM, Toppari J, Skakkebæk NE. Testicular descent: INSL3, testosterone, genes and the intrauterine milieu. Nature Reviews Urology. 2011;**8**(4):187-196

[13] Ferlin A. Genetic alterations associated with cryptorchidism. Journal of the American Medical Association. 2008;**300**(19):2271

[14] Rodprasert W, Virtanen HE, Mäkelä JA, Toppari J. Hypogonadism and cryptorchidism. Frontiers in Endocrinology. 2020;**10**:906

[15] Kalfa N, Gaspari L, Ollivier M, Philibert P, Bergougnoux A, Paris F, et al. Molecular genetics of hypospadias and cryptorchidism recent developments. Clinical Genetics [Internet]. 2019;**95**(1):122-131. Available from: https://pubmed.ncbi.nlm.nih.gov/30084162/

[16] Barthold JS, Wang Y, Kolon TF, Kollin C, Nordenskjöld A, Olivant

Fisher A, et al. Pathway analysis supports association of nonsyndromic cryptorchidism with genetic loci linked to cytoskeleton-dependent functions. Human Reproduction [Internet]. 2015;**30**(10):2439-2451. Available from: https://pubmed.ncbi.nlm.nih.gov/26209787/

[17] Zimmermann S, Steding G, Emmen JMA, Brinkmann AO, Nayernia K, Holstein AF, et al. Targeted disruption of the Insl3 gene causes bilateral cryptorchidism. Molecular Endocrinology [Internet]. 1999;**13**(5):681-691. Available from: https://academic.oup.com/mend/article/13/5/681/2741612

[18] Ferlin A. Insulin-like factor 3 gene mutations in testicular dysgenesis syndrome: Clinical and functional characterization. Molecular Human Reproduction [Internet]. 2006;**12**(6):401-406. Available from: https://academic.oup.com/molehr/article-abstract/12/6/401/1044750?redirectedFrom=fulltext&login=false

[19] McElreavey K, Jorgensen A, Eozenou C, Merel T, Bignon-Topalovic J, Tan DS, et al. Pathogenic variants in the DEAH-box RNA helicase DHX37 are a frequent cause of 46,XY gonadal dysgenesis and 46,XY testicular regression syndrome. Genetics in Medicine [Internet]. 2019;**22**(1):150-159. Available from: https://www.nature.com/articles/s41436-019-0606-y

[20] Wang Q, Ge X, Wang HX, Shi QM, Ding Z, Xu LC. Association of androgen receptor gene CAG and GGN repeat polymorphism with cryptorchidism: A meta-analysis. Andrologia [Internet]. 2017;**50**(3):e12909-e12909 Available from: https://pubmed.ncbi.nlm.nih.gov/29044734/

[21] Hughes IA, Davies JD, Bunch TI, Pasterski V, Mastroyannopoulou K, MacDougall J. Androgen insensitivity syndrome. Lancet (London, England) [Internet]. 2012;**380**(9851):1419-1428. Available from: https://www.ncbi.nlm.nih.gov/pubmed/22698698

[22] Capra AP, Ferro E, Angela M, Briuglia S, Russo T, Arena S, et al. Genetic analysis of the human insulin-like 3 gene in pediatric patients with testicular torsion. Pediatric Surgery International [Internet]. 2018;**34**(7):807-812. Available from: https://pubmed.ncbi.nlm.nih.gov/29785651/

[23] Hutson JM, Thorup JM, Beasley SW. Descent of the Testis. 2nd ed. New York Dordrecht London: Cham Springer International Publishing; 2016

[24] Virtanen HE, Bjerknes R, Cortes D, Jørgensen N, Rajpert-De Meyts E, Thorsson AV, et al. Cryptorchidism: Classification, prevalence and long-term consequences. Acta Paediatrica. 2007;**96**(5):611-616

[25] AbouZeid AA, Mousa MH, Soliman HA, Hamza AF, Hay SA. Intra-abdominal testis: Histological alterations and significance of biopsy. The Journal of Urology [Internet]. 2011;**185**(1):269-274. DOI: 10.1016/j.juro.2010.09.026?utm_source=chatgpt.com

[26] Sepúlveda X, Egaña PJL. Current management of non-palpable testes: A literature review and clinical results. Translational Pediatrics. 2017;**5**(4):233-239

[27] American Urological Association. Evaluation and Treatment of Cryptorchidism (2018) [Internet]. Linthicum, MD: American Urological Association; 2018. Available from: https://www.auanet.org/guidelines-and-quality/guidelines/cryptorchidism-guideline

[28] Ayhan A, Gönül Ç, Ahmet A, Ece B. Epidemiology, classification and management of undescended testes: Does medication have value in its treatment? Journal of Clinical Research in Pediatric Endocrinology [Internet]. 2013;**5**(2):65-72. DOI: 10.4274%2FJcrpe.883

[29] Merry C, Sweeney B, Puri P. The vanishing testis: Anatomical and histological findings. European Urology. 1997;**31**(1):65-67

[30] Yeap E, Nataraja RM, Pacilli M. Undescended testes: What general practitioners need to know. Australian Journal of General Practice [Internet]. 2019;**48**(1-2):33-36. Available from: https://www1.racgp.org.au/ajgp/2019/january%E2%80%93february/undescended-testes?utm_source=chatgpt.com

[31] Docimo SG, Silver RI, Cromie W. The undescended testicle: Diagnosis and management. American Family Physician [Internet]. 2000;**62**(9):2037-2044. Available from: https://www.aafp.org/pubs/afp/issues/2000/1101/p2037.html?utm_source=chatgpt.com

[32] Shin J, Jeon GW. Comparison of diagnostic and treatment guidelines for undescended testis. Clinical and Experimental Pediatrics. 2020;**63**(11):415-421

[33] Kolon TF, Herndon CDA, Baker LA, Baskin LS, Baxter CG, Cheng EY, et al. Evaluation and treatment of cryptorchidism: AUA guideline. Journal of Urology. 2014;**192**(2):337-345

[34] Tasian GE, Copp HL. Diagnostic performance of ultrasound in nonpalpable cryptorchidism: A systematic review and meta-analysis. Pediatrics [Internet]. 2010;**127**(1):119-128. Available from: https://pubmed.ncbi.nlm.nih.gov/21149435/

[35] Krishnaswami S, Fonnesbeck C, Penson D, McPheeters ML. Magnetic resonance imaging for locating nonpalpable undescended testicles: A meta-analysis. Pediatrics. 2013;**131**(6):e1908-e1916

[36] Berger C, Haid B, Becker T, Koen M, Roesch J, Oswald J. Nonpalpable testes: Ultrasound and contralateral testicular hypertrophy predict the surgical access, avoiding unnecessary laparoscopy. Journal of Pediatric Urology. 2018;**14**(2):163.e1-163.e7

[37] Niedzielski JK, Oszukowska E, Słowikowska-Hilczer J. Undescended testis – Current trends and guidelines: A review of the literature. Archives of Medical Science. 2016;**3**(12):667-677

[38] Hay SA, Soliman HA, Abdel AH, Bassiouny IE. Laparoscopic classification and treatment of the impalpable testis. Pediatric Surgery International [Internet]. 1999;**15**(8):570-572. Available from: https://pubmed.ncbi.nlm.nih.gov/10631737/

[39] Mayo Clinic. Undescended Testicle – Diagnosis and Treatment [Internet]. Rochester, MN: Mayo Clinic; 2019. Available from: https://www.mayoclinic.org/diseases-conditions/undescended-testicle/diagnosis-treatment/drc-20352000

[40] Pakkasjärvi N, Taskinen S. Surgical treatment of cryptorchidism: Current insights and future directions. Frontiers in Endocrinology. 2024;**15**:1327957. Available from: https://www.ncbi.nlm.nih.gov/pmc/articles/PMC10940471/pdf/fendo-15-1327957.pdf

[41] Errico A, Ambrosini G, Vinco S, Bottani E, Pozza ED, Marroncelli N, et al. In vitro effect of hCG on cryptorchid patients' gubernacular cells: A predictive model for adjuvant personalized

therapy. Cell Communication and Signaling [Internet]. 2025;**23**(1):1327957. DOI: 10.1186/s12964-024-01979-y

[42] Chung E, Brock GB. Cryptorchidism and its impact on male fertility: A state of art review of current literature. Canadian Urological Association Journal = Journal de l'Association des urologues du Canada [Internet]. 2011;**5**(3):210-214. Available from: https://www.ncbi.nlm.nih.gov/pmc/articles/PMC3114036/

[43] Rodprasert W, Virtanen HE, Mäkelä JA, Toppari J. Hypogonadism and cryptorchidism. Frontiers in Endocrinology [Internet]. 2020;**10**:906. Available from: https://pmc.ncbi.nlm.nih.gov/articles/PMC6974459/

[44] Hadžiselimović F, Verkauskas G, Stadler M. Epigenetics, cryptorchidism, and infertility. Basic and Clinical Andrology [Internet]. 2023;**33**:1. DOI: 10.1186/s12610-023-00199-7

[45] Kano T, Kojima T, Takahashi T, Muto Y. Serum thyroid hormone levels in patients with fulminant hepatitis: Usefulness of rT3 and the rT3/T3 ratio as prognostic indices. Gastroenterologia Japonica [Internet]. 1987;**22**(3):344-353. Available from: https://pubmed.ncbi.nlm.nih.gov/3114036/

[46] Holder J, Binet E, Flanigan S, Ferris E. Arteriography after carotid endarterectomy. American Journal of Roentgenology [Internet]. 1981;**137**(3):483-487. Available from: https://pubmed.ncbi.nlm.nih.gov/6974459/

[47] Avakoudjo J, Hodonou F, Sewa EV, Tandje Y, Sossa J, Yevi M, et al. Undescended testis in adult: Epidemiology and therapeutic aspects. About 23 cases in HKM university teaching Hospital of Cotonou. Open Journal of Urology [Internet]. 2018;**08**(07):206-213. Available from: https://www.scirp.org/journal/paperinformation?paperid=86208

[48] Viljoen JT, Zarrabi A, Van der Merwe A. Management of cryptorchidism in adolescent and adult males. African Journal of Urology [Internet]. 2020;**26**:1. Available from: https://afju.springeropen.com/articles/10.1186/s12301-020-00051-8#citeas

[49] Jeong SC, Lee S, Ku JY, Lee SD. Clinical characteristics and treatment of cryptorchidism in adults: A single center experience. The World Journal of Men's Health [Internet]. 2014;**32**(2):110. DOI: 10.5534/wjmh.2014.32.2.110

[50] Ates F, Soydan H, Okcelik S, Cirakoglu A, Yilmaz I, Malkoc E, et al. Clinical and histopathological results of the adult patients with unilateral cryptorchidism patients. Türk Üroloji Dergisi/Turkish Journal of Urology [Internet]. 2016;**42**(2):74-79. Available from: https://www.urologyresearchandpractice.org/en/clinical-and-histopathological-results-of-the-adult-patients-with-unilateral-cryptorchidism-132923

[51] Li J, Zhou L, Huang S, Duan T, Xie J, Li X, et al. The effect of endocrine-disrupting chemicals in follicular fluid: The insights from oocyte to fertilization. Environment International [Internet]. 2024;**191**:108957-108957. Available from: https://www.sciencedirect.com/science/article/pii/S0160412024005439

[52] Constâncio V, Tavares NT, Henrique R, Jerónimo C, Lobo J. MiRNA biomarkers in cancers of the male reproductive system: Are we approaching clinical application? Andrology [Internet]. 2022;**11**(4):651-667. DOI: 10.1111/andr.13258

[53] Pettersson A, Richiardi L, Nordenskjold A, Kaijser M, Akre O.